How To Be

HEALTH STRONG

WHAT YOUR DOCTOR
DIDN'T TELL YOU

How To Be
HEALTH STRONG

WHAT YOUR DOCTOR DIDN'T TELL YOU

A Complete Guide to Building an
Armor-Like Immune System to Live
Longer and Feel Younger
... at Any Age!

Robert Louis Drapkin, MD, FACP
Donny Kim, Master Trainer, PES, CPT-NASM

Editing: Writer Services, LLC (WriterServices.net)
Cover Design & Book Layout: Writer Services, LLC

ISBN 13: 978-1-942389-26-2

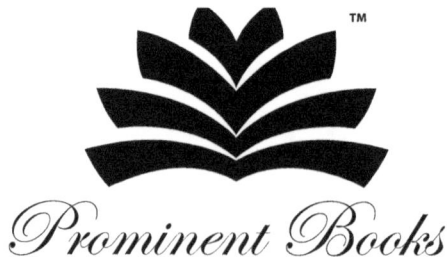

Prominent Books

TABLE OF CONTENTS

DISCLAIMER

The publisher and the author are providing this book and its contents on an "as is" basis and make no representations or warranties of any kind with respect to this book or its contents. The publisher and the author disclaim all such representations and warranties, including but not limited to warranties of healthcare for a particular purpose. In addition, the publisher and the author assume no responsibility for errors, inaccuracies, omissions, or any other inconsistencies herein.

The content of this book is for informational purposes only and is not intended to diagnose, treat, cure, or prevent any condition or disease. You understand that this book is not intended as a substitute for consultation with a licensed practitioner. Please consult with your own physician or healthcare specialist regarding the suggestions and recommendations made in this book. The use of this book implies your acceptance of this disclaimer.

The publisher and the author make no guarantees concerning the level of success you may experience by following the advice and strategies contained in this book, and you accept the risk that results will differ for each individual. The testimonials and examples provided in this book show exceptional results, which may not apply to the average reader, and are not intended to represent or guarantee that you will achieve the same or similar results.

THE OPTIMAL BODY

CHAPTER 1
The Most Important Thing

Most Americans today are unhealthy. Most Americans do not know what is healthy to eat, what is healthy to drink, and how to keep the body healthy. Do you have too much belly fat? Do you have five alcoholic drinks each week? Do you exercise? Do you eat fast food? Do you sleep well? How is your sex life? Most medical doctors today are no better than you. They do not have the training needed to keep you healthy and to prevent the most common occurring diseases. Doctors are trained to treat the sick, not to prevent illness. I know this because I was guilty of this. Most Americans do not have a healthy lifestyle—that means you—and it is not your fault. This book is the answer, and anyone can improve.

This text is based upon science, and most statements have a reference to the scientific literature. The purpose of this book is to take what is published in the most up-to-date scientific journals and introduce this knowledge into your everyday life to make your life better.

We will train you like an athlete in the contest of your life.

The first thing we will do is convince you that most Americans (and many people in the world) are not healthy. We will then explain how your body works. We will tell you about food,

1

exercise, supplements, hormone replacement therapy, and provide a roadmap toward good health. This is a path for a healthy life. If it were a race, it would be the race won by the turtle—one small step in the right direction every day.

Why We Wrote This Book

I'm unhappy with the medical culture in the United States because it focuses on treating the symptoms of the sick and does little to prevent the most common chronic diseases that are the leading causes of death and disability—**and which are completely preventable!** If you don't have the knowledge contained in this book, you'll likely develop a chronic metabolic illness, and you'll be given prescription medications and likely told that it's part of "growing old" when, in fact, **it is *not*.**

The Centers for Disease Control and Prevention (CDC) clearly attests to this statement: lack of exercise, poor nutrition, tobacco use and alcohol cause much of the current chronic metabolic diseases, pain, and early deaths [1-3]. These chronic metabolic diseases (hypertension, stroke, type 2 diabetes, coronary artery disease, dementia) are the leading causes of death and disability in the United States [4]. Most adults do not follow the CDC's recommendations. Modern primary care physicians are trained to treat these same metabolic problems—hypertension, adult-onset insulin resistant (type 2) diabetes, erectile dysfunction, coronary artery disease, stroke and dementia. **Most physicians do not provide detailed information on how to *prevent* these diseases—and this is truly the most important medical knowledge that everyone needs to have!** Has your physician told you to lose weight but did not give you a specific diet plan tailored to your needs? Did your physician give you a diet and exercise program? **Did your physician just give you pills?**

Most patients today accept the minimal advice that their family doctors and nurse practitioners give them: **LOSE WEIGHT, AND EXERCISE.** Most patients take some of the pills prescribed to them, and that is all they do. These medications—such as metformin, metoprolol and atorvastatin—are good medications, but they do not cure diseases. These pills palliate (lessen the severity of) diseases by hiding the signs of disease, giving patients a false sense of security and telling them that they can continue to live their unhealthy lifestyle. It's "OK" because "I take my blood pressure medication, my cholesterol medication, and my pills for my elevated glucose." The proof of the disconnect between pills, doctor advice, and health was recently published in the British Journal of Pharmacology [5]. High blood pressure is perhaps the most common condition treated by medication in a primary care medical office. It is well known that people with high blood pressure are at higher risk for cardiovascular complications than people without high blood pressure, and this is not controversial [6]. The real question remains, does treatment of high blood pressure with medication reduce the risk of cardiovascular disease? The answer to this is, unfortunately, **not always**. Blood pressure medication lowers the blood pressure, but the causes of most adult onset hypertension remain in place—an unhealthy lifestyle, and the heart disease continues to develop [6].

The most difficult challenge today is *changing* **your lifestyle and** *eliminating the need* **for these pills**. The average American over 18 years of age fills twelve different prescriptions each year and takes over ten pills per day [7]. How many do you take?

The real benefit to lifestyle change is the removal of hypertension, insulin-resistant diabetes, and vascular diseases. And more importantly, you'll live longer and feel stronger. Every organ in your body, including your brain, will perform better. Yes, even your sex life will improve.

I'm impressed with people who pay meticulous attention to their clothing. I'm impressed with the people who maintain their auto-mobiles in spotless condition. I'm impressed with apartments and homes that have beautiful rooms and furniture. Why do we not pay meticulous attention to our bodies?

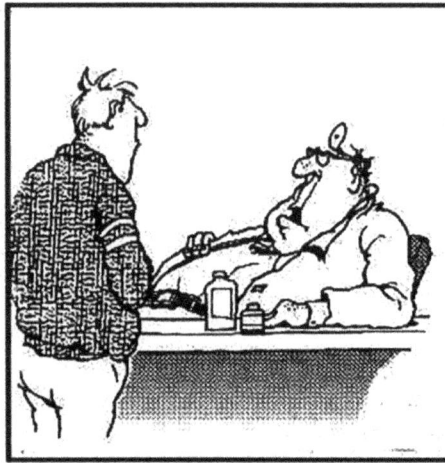

"Are you eating properly and getting plenty of exercise?"

This is a reference book. You do not need to read every sentence. The main points are stated in the beginning of each chapter. The scientific terms and medical terms are in *italics* and [brackets] and may be skipped if you wish. Every statement is referenced for those who wish to read the primary sources.

CHAPTER 2
Americans Are Unhealthy— Sicker Than Any Other Industrialized Country

According to the Mayo Clinic, over 97% of Americans are unhealthy and at increased risk for cardiovascular disease and type 2 diabetes chronic metabolic illnesses [1]. These Mayo supported researchers studied 4,745 people in regard to diet, exercise, smoking, and body fat. The authors used objective measures of health and did not rely solely on subjective patient surveys.

[Measurements of exercise were performed using an accelerometer, with a healthy goal of 150 minutes of moderate to vigorous exercise per week. Blood pressure was measured with a standard blood monitor and cuff in mm of mercury. Blood tests were performed to measure: evidence of smoking, C-reactive protein, lipid profiles, glucose, and homocysteine. Body fat was not calculated but measured accurately using X-ray absorptiometry (DXA or DEXA). A healthy diet was defined by the USDA.]

The results: 71% did not smoke; 38% ate a healthy diet; 10% had a normal body fat percentage; 46% had sufficient exercise; and only 2.7% had all four healthy measurements.

Recent data estimates that 38% of adults and 15% to 20% of children in the USA are obese [2, 8]. Obesity is a major risk factor for a heart attack or myocardial infarction [3].

According to the National Center for Health Statistics, we are getting sicker. Life expectancy in the USA has decreased for the second time in 21 years, to 78.6 years from 78.9 years [6]. A small decrease, but a sign of increasing chronic metabolic disease: heart disease, stroke, Alzheimer's Disease, and diabetes. Compared to 35 industrialized countries, the USA ranks 26th in life expectancy [4]. Japan leads the list with an average life expectancy of 84 years, and nearly all western European countries do better than the USA. The research council of the U.S. Institute of Medicine reported that cardiovascular diseases in industrialized countries have declined everywhere except in the United States. **In summary, Americans live shorter lives than people in any other high-income country [5] and are the fattest adults in the world [7].**

Mr. B's Story

Mr. B was born and raised in Chicago. He worked hard all his life and finally retired at age 65 and moved to Florida. When I first met Mr. B, his chief complaints were fatigue, no sex life, and weakness. His past medical history included high blood pressure, coronary artery disease with a stent placement, and poorly controlled adult-onset (type 2) diabetes. His medications included metformin and insulin for his diabetes and a statin. He took two medications for his high blood pressure and an anticoagulant. He saw his cardiologist and primary care physician on a regular basis.

On physical exam, his initial blood pressure was elevated at 169/98, and he weighed 226 pounds, with a BMI of 32, and was thus obese. His physical exam was otherwise normal except for slight swelling in both lower extremities. Blood tests showed that his blood sugar was elevated at 160 mg/dl, despite his medications for diabetes, and he had mild kidney damage (creatinine 1.3/GFR 50ml/minute). His waist-to-height ratio was 40/68, or 0.58, and revealed an increased risk for cardiovascular disease [9].

In summary, Mr. B had measurable disease caused by his unhealthy lifestyle that persisted despite his medical intervention with pills and injections. Furthermore, he had low testosterone levels and thus had testicular hypofunction.

Mr. B ate most of his meals at fast food restaurants—his favorite was Taco Bell®. He snacked on candy bars despite his diabetes. He had not done any exercising since high school. He did take all his medications and felt secure that he was medically well despite his dysfunctions. He asked me what I recommended.

I told Mr. B that he needed to lose body fat and that this could best be done with a lower calorie diet that is higher in protein and fat, along with eliminating high sugar-containing foods, averaging 1,600 calories—approximately 500 calories below his daily needs. I also found a personal trainer for Mr. B, and he started to exercise. I told him that if he could lose one pound per week and exercise three hours per week, then, after four weeks, I would consider prescribing supplements to return his low testosterone levels to normal.

After four weeks, Mr. B had made no progress whatsoever. He couldn't change his eating habits or lifestyle, and he quit the gym.

One year later, he came back to my office after having suffered a heart attack (myocardial infarction). His problems had increased despite the medications he'd been taking. He again asked me what to do, and I simply said, "What you're doing now is not working! If you don't change, you'll continue to get worse."

We'll try again to help Mr. B and prevent further organ damage with diet and exercise to prolong his life. Interestingly, he drives a meticulously maintained eight-year-old car that looks brand new and lives in a perfectly maintained model home. His health is his most valuable possession, yet it is in poor condition.

Signs Your Body Needs Help

You have difficulty falling asleep. This is likely due to stress in your life and the subsequent elevation of the stress hormone, cortisol. Sleep is your body's method of recovering from daily stress, but if the stress is too great, cortisol levels remain high, and insomnia results. There are three possible solutions: one, to resolve the issues causing the stress; two, to relieve the stress through exercise, which lowers cortisol levels; or three, take a sleeping pill.

The stress-inducing issues may take a long time to resolve. Exercise is therefore the best option, since it solves the problem quickly. Developing a pill habit leads to more potential complications. Some people do benefit from short-acting sleep aids that are prescribed only as needed.

You are getting shorter. Your height decreases because your bones are losing calcium due to a dietary lack of calcium (poor nutrition) or a Vitamin D deficiency. These nutritional deficiencies allow your spinal bones to flatten (compression fractures). Adult height loss can also be caused by curvature of the spine (kyphosis), which is due to nutritional deficiencies as noted above, as well as muscle weakness. A hormone deficiency is a common cause of bone density loss, and this can be corrected with hormone replacement therapy. Has your doctor checked all your hormone levels?

Your body is shaped like an apple, with your abdominal girth (waist size) bigger than your hip measurements. Visceral body fat is the fat that accumulates around your internal abdominal organs and increases the size of your waist. A waist-to-height ratio greater than 0.5 is a simple and accurate predictor of heart disease risk. This problem can be solved with both diet and exercise used together.

You have little energy. Fatigue can be caused by a variety of problems, such as low thyroid, low testosterone, poor nutrition, and/or abnormal metabolism. Your brain can decrease your metabolic rate. This is a complex problem that can be handled with diet, exercise, and the use of appropriate supplements as discussed later in this book. This is also a symptom of possible sleep apnea. If you snore and are tired all day, you likely have sleep apnea. This is a condition in which the fatty tissues of your body obstruct air flow into your lungs while you sleep, causing a lower oxygen level in your blood and body. This can be cured with loss of body fat. Most doctors palliate this with a wearable medical device that increases air flow, called a CPAP machine. The CPAP works well but never cures the problem.

My Story—What's in This for You?

The purpose of this book is to provide you with all the knowledge you'll need in order to improve your health and obtain the strength, vigor, and muscular body you once had (or wish to have). This text is a roadmap to good health and can take you beyond your expectations. I expect that since you're reading this, you're dissatisfied with your current body shape, and you wish to do something about it. I was in your shoes at 48 years of age, and I had no idea how to change my life and become healthy despite my medical training. Medical school does not teach the essentials of diet and exercise as medical treatments to prevent disease. Medical school teaches how to treat disease.

What was happening to me in my forties has (or will) happen to you. I thought I knew how to eat healthy food and how to exercise. I thought I looked good. My wife and I went on vacation to Cozumel, Mexico. We rented a Jeep so we could go exploring and take photographs. In those days, we used film cameras and had to wait for the film to be developed before we could see the pictures.

Below is a picture of me during that vacation at age 48.

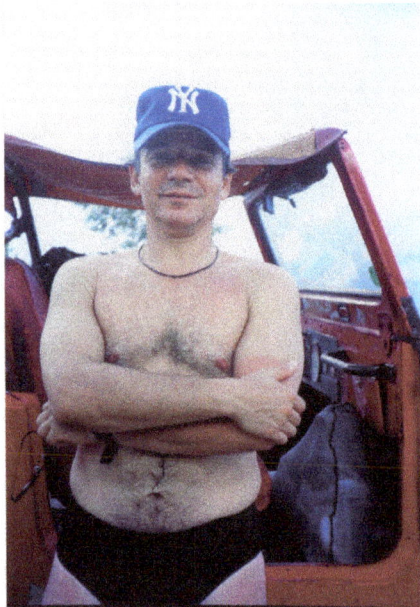

Robert Drapkin, Age 48

What's humorous about this is that I'd thought I looked good, until the photo arrived, at which time I saw myself with a potbelly, a double chin, and a ridiculous attitude. This image was the stimulus for me to join a gym and restart my education with diet and exercise.

I joined a gym and attempted to work out on my own, as I was a physician and thought I knew everything. In reality, I knew nothing, and for over two years, my body didn't change—my love handles stayed put, along with my double chin.

Then, by chance, I met Donny Kim, a certified personal trainer with a special interest in body mechanics and a champion body-builder. Donny started me on the road to good health, fitness, and strength. We've remained good friends for 20 years, and now we decided to put in writing all the knowledge we've learned on how to transform adults—both male and female—into strong, healthy, and robust human beings.

If you decide to follow this roadmap, you'll feel the difference within three weeks and see the difference within three months. Please take a photograph of yourself right now, get on the scale and weigh yourself, and measure your waist with a tape measure. Write down these numbers or store these data points on your mobile phone, and date the photograph. If your waist in inches divided by your height in inches is greater than 0.5, you are very unhealthy. If you're unhappy with this photo and the numbers, you've just started on your road back to good health!

Below is an image of me at age 66—18 years later:

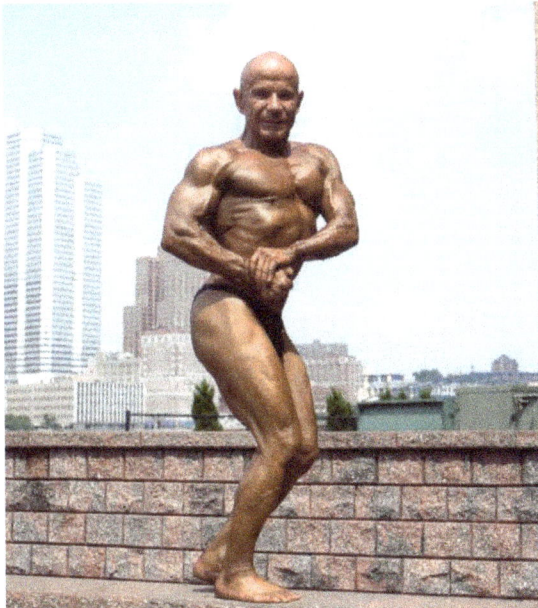

CHAPTER 3
Long-Term Behavioral Change

There are three essential components to long-term behavioral change [1]:

1. You must have a goal;

2. You must be able to measure your progress; and

3. You must have willpower.

Willpower is the ability to postpone instant gratification in order to achieve a long-term goal. This involves the ability to control your impulses. Impulsivity involves an action that occurs with little or no planning or thinking, as opposed to actions that require careful thinking towards a planned outcome. The classic marshmallow experiment [2] showed that children able to delay gratification—one marshmallow now versus two marshmallows later—grew to be healthier and more successful adults. There are simple things you can do to increase your willpower:

1. Take slow, deep diaphragmatic breaths lasting 10 to 15 seconds per breath, which will decrease heart rate variability before you act [3, 4].

2. Increase exercise [5].

3. Work with successful people who have similar goals [6, 7].

4. Wait for 10 minutes before acting—change fast thinking to slow contemplation [8].

5. Think about your goals [8].

How Your Brain Works—Decision-Making and Willpower

[The process of decision-making depends on the parts of the brain that regulate emotion and feeling and the neurotransmitters serotonin and dopamine.

Both the amygdala and the ventromedial prefrontal cortex [VMPC] are the crucial parts of the brain for decision-making. The amygdala responds to everything that occurs in the environment, whereas the VMPC triggers emotions and somatic states from memories and knowledge.

Willpower emerges from the dynamic interaction of these two separate brain areas. The amygdala is a critical neural structure involved in triggering the fast-affective/emotional signals of immediate thinking and actions. The VMPC is a critical neural structure involved in triggering the slower reflective-affective/emotional signals of long-term outcomes and plans.

Willpower uses the VMPC. So go slow, and you will be in control.]

CHAPTER 4
How We Get Fat—Sugar Addiction

High sugar containing foods [high glycemic] are different than any other foods. High sugar foods stimulate the addiction center of the brain. This is the region of the brain called the nucleus accumbens (NA). Low sugar containing foods do not do this. The NA is the pleasure center or reward center of the brain. **Both high sugar containing foods and addictive drugs such as heroin cause dopamine release into the NA.** This can be measured by brain imaging scans that light up the NA, and human subjects report euphoria or a high [1].

Daily bingeing on high sugar foods repeatedly releases dopamine in the nucleus accumbens. This is how we become addicted to sugar or any other food or substance such as pain medication. **Sugar is actually more addictive than cocaine [2, 3].**

Why is Sugar a Problem?

Sugar or anything that tastes sweet will increase blood sugar, causing insulin release from the pancreas. Insulin is the fat storage hormone. Insulin lowers your blood sugar level to normal and stores this excess sugar as body fat. Insulin makes body fat.

Sugar in our food is the reason over 60% of Americans are overweight or obese, and any food that raises your insulin levels is addictive.

The body fat around your belly—visceral body fat—produces inflammatory molecules that damage small blood vessels, ultimately resulting in hypertension, type 2 diabetes, coronary artery (heart) disease, dementia, impotence, and kidney and liver dysfunction. In addition, in the presence of high insulin levels, your body is unable to know when to stop eating. The body's feedback mechanism to stop eating is the release of leptin by fat cells, which tells your brain you have enough food, and the brain stops producing the hunger hormone ghrelin. If insulin is high, the feedback loop is blocked, and the brain continues to produce ghrelin. You are hungry despite having enough stored food, so you eat more and get fat.

The large food companies have added sweeteners—sugar, fructose, artificial sweeteners—to packaged foods in order to sell more food products. In addition, these same companies spend large sums of money to market these unhealthy food products.

Normal Control of Food Intake—
Low Glycemic Food, Normal Insulin Level

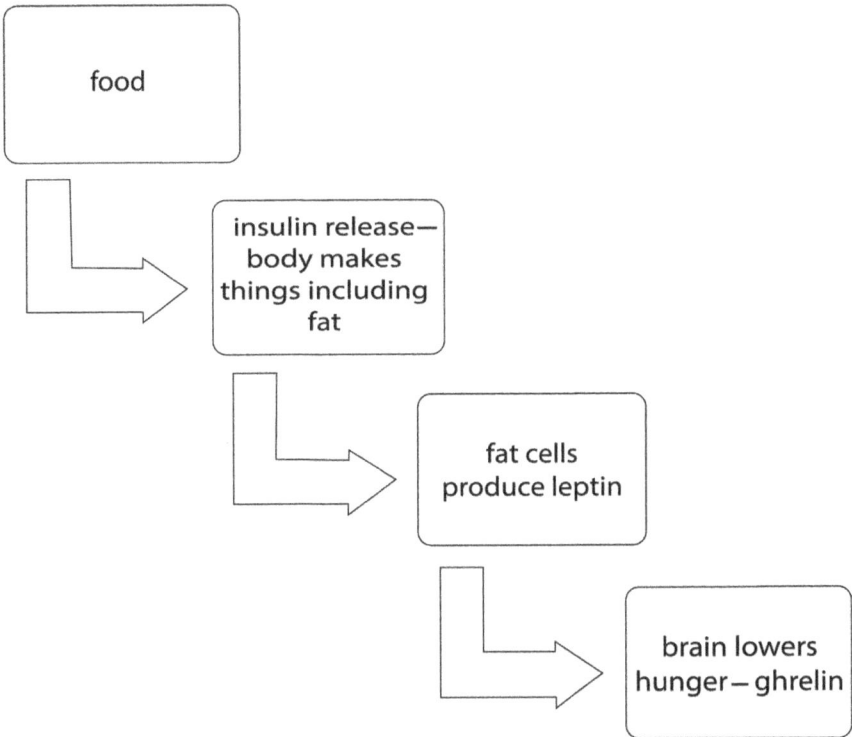

food

→ insulin release—body makes things including fat

→ fat cells produce leptin

→ brain lowers hunger—ghrelin

How We Get Fat—
Leptin Blocked By High Insulin

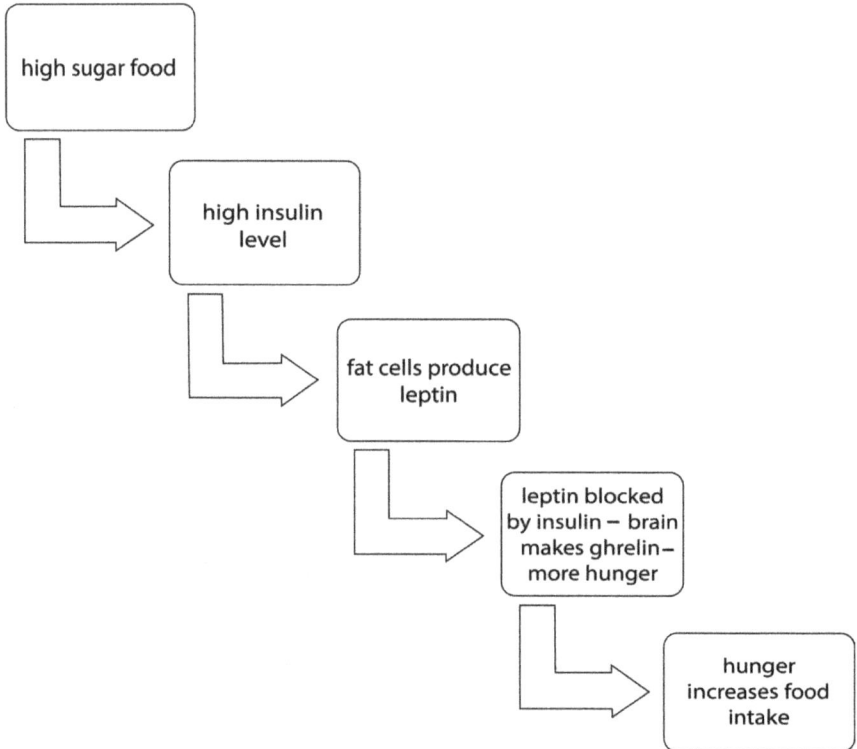

high sugar food

high insulin level

fat cells produce leptin

leptin blocked by insulin – brain makes ghrelin– more hunger

hunger increases food intake

The above explanation is a simplified version of the complex interaction between the brain and the hormones/peptides that increase and decrease hunger. The hunger hormones/peptides made in the brain (hypothalamus) that stimulate feeding include NPY and AgRP. The stomach peptide ghrelin increases hunger by stimulating NPY and AgRP and blocking leptin.

The brain peptides that decrease hunger and increase metabolic rate include POMC/a-MSH and CART. To decrease hunger, the duodenum and small intestine produce CCK, the intestines produce PYY, and the pancreas produces PP. The intestines produce Oxynto-modulin and GLP-1 to decrease GI motility, the pancreas produces Insulin, and fat cells produce Leptin and Adiponectin. Leptin inhibits NPY, AgRP and stimulates POMC and CART. Leptin is a major player in appetite reduction [4].

There is new data that some processed foods contain chemicals that cause insulin resistance and hunger, and this is discussed in chapter nine on diet.

CHAPTER 5
Age Can Change Your Body

We are born, we develop, we decline, and we die. The purpose of this book is to prolong the *develop* and delay the *decline* by understanding how your body works. The most important aspect of good health and longevity is knowledge. The first part of this book will increase your understanding of how your body works. The next part of this book will outline the actions or the things you can accomplish with diet and exercise. This includes the path to building muscle, lowering body fat, and increasing energy. The third subjects you will learn about are supplements, medical weight loss, and hormones. Once you have this knowledge, you can create your own healthy lifestyle. We inherit the genes of our parents, and we learn from our parents what to eat. We mimic their lifestyle (at least in early life). To improve, we need to learn from their mistakes and avail ourselves of more recently discovered information. Our tool kit includes diet, exercise, and supplements/hormones/peptides. **If you wish to have your Optimal Body, you will need to use all the tools in your tool kit.**

Today, there is an epidemic of obesity, leading to an epidemic of metabolic diseases. The National Institute of Health found that in 2009-2010, two out of three adults were overweight with a BMI of 25-29.9; one out of three adults were obese with a BMI of 30-39.9; and one out of twenty adults were morbidly obese with a BMI of 40+ [1].

Morbid obesity is defined as a BMI greater than 40 and refers to a body that has medical problems due specifically to excess body fat. All of these problems can be prevented or lessened by using the knowledge presented in this book. Modern medicine prefers to palliate metabolic syndrome, hypertension, insulin-resistant diabetes, and hyperlipidemia with drugs. Yet if you're motivated to learn from this book and understand your body, you'll enjoy a longer, healthier, and more energetic life.

There are eight common changes in your body that occur between the ages of 40 and 60 in addition to those changes associated with metabolic changes. These eight changes are familiar to all, and all can be treated or improved with diet, exercise, and supplements. Memory loss [2]; bone and joint pain [3]; vision loss [4]; loss of skin elasticity [5]; frailty or muscular weakness due to muscle loss [7]; loss of sexual function/interest [12, 7]; increase in body fat [8]; and loss of bone density [6].

Memory. Exercise will help to improve your memory [2]. In the elderly, the memory part of the brain—the hippocampus—shrinks as memory decreases. Exercise and nutrition increase the size of the hippocampus and cause memory improvement, thus reversing the effects of aging.

Bone and joint pain. Obesity associated with aging is also significantly associated with increased osteoarthritis of the knees due to the increased mechanical stress placed on the knees by increased body fat and the compensatory alterations in body mechanics [3]. By losing body fat, you can regain a normal gait pattern ("gait" is the way you walk), and your knee pain will decrease. Strengthening core muscles is essential in eliminating lower back pain. Exercise and core muscle strength eliminate the need for back and knee surgery if started before serious damage occurs.

Vision loss. Visual field loss is associated strongly with decreased mobility [4]. Another aspect of vision loss is small blood vessel damage associated with diabetes, and insulin resistance caused by obesity and a sedentary lifestyle. If you prevent insulin resistance and prevent diabetes (as outlined in this book), you can save your vision.

Loss of skin elasticity. We start losing muscle mass at age 30+, and we become weaker, more sedentary, and gain body fat. As growth hormones, androgen and estrogen levels diminish with age, we lose tissue elasticity, and wrinkles increase [5]. Exercise and supplements are able to restore these hormone levels to normal values, thus reversing skin elasticity. Your wrinkles will disappear, and your skin will tighten back up. You won't need plastic surgery.

Loss of muscle mass and increase in body fat. Body fat increases with age as you lose muscle mass. You lose approximately 1% of muscle mass each year starting in your thirties, and by age 60, it's possible to have lost 30% of muscle tissue. With less muscle, you will do less activity and retain body fat [7, 8].

Loss of sexual function/interest. Loss of sexual interest and performance is a complicated issue involving multiple organ systems. Suffice it to say, exercise, diet, and supplements will raise sex hormone levels to their normal ranges [12]. If a hormone deficiency is the cause of the problem, this can be cured with hormone replacement therapy in both men and women.

Loss of bone density. As you age, bone density decreases, and you become shorter. Bone loss with age is common. Bone mass peaks at ages 25-30 and then decreases slowly in both men and women [6]. The amount of bone loss in the elderly is determined by many factors including diet, exercise, calcium, vitamin D, nutrition, hormone levels, gender, and genetics. Women have more rapid bone loss than men during their post-menopausal years. Postmenopausal women also have a higher incidence of bone fracture than do men. Bone density is easily measured by a test called a dual-energy X-ray absorptiometry (DEXA or DXA) bone density scan. This procedure is described in the next section of this book.

A DEXA scan will directly measure bone mineral density (BMD) and tell you a number (Tscore). If your Tscore is slightly below normal (1 to 2.5 standard deviations), you have osteopenia (mildly reduced bone mass) and need to take vitamin D and possibly calcium supplements, as well as increase your physical activity. If your Tscore is low (2.5 standard deviations from normal), you're at higher risk of bone fractures, and you need to take not only vitamin D and calcium but an additional medication (usually a bisphosphonate). You also may need hormone replacement therapy, which in post-menopausal women is the most likely cause of bone density loss. *Bisphosphonates prevent calcium loss in bones by blocking the cells (osteoclasts) that resorb bone.* Exercise also prevents bone density loss but only in the presence of normal hormone levels. The purpose of these treatments is to prevent bone fractures. The bisphosphonates have been well studied in expensive, prospective, randomized studies paid for by the drug companies and do prevent bone fractures. Bisphosphonates are patented drugs that have been profitable for the drug makers and justify the expensive clinical trials. Bisphosphonates are preferred by many doctors over hormone replacement because of the lack of data regarding fracture prevention with hormone replacement. **The simple truth is, hormone replacement with bioidentical estrogen or testosterone will never be studied in fracture prevention because they cannot be patented and will never be profitable enough to pay for the clinical trials.** This is a good example of how profitable, patented, expensive drugs have replaced hormone replacement therapy in a medical condition often caused by a hormone deficiency.

John T's Story

John was a 50-year-old car salesman. He had been very successful in his career but noticed that his younger competitors were becoming more successful. He had difficulty remembering customers' names. He noticed an increase in his waist size, and his shirts were tight around his neck. In the mornings, his knees hurt. He called this his *football knees*. He began ending each day drinking scotch and smoking to better control the stress in his life. He lost interest in sex due to his inability to perform. Even though he played varsity football in high school and understood the value of exercise, he hadn't exercised in 30 years. His diet consisted of fast food for breakfast and lunch and bar food for dinner. While driving home one evening, he was involved in a motor vehicle accident and injured his neck and lower back. His doctor told him he had compression fractures in his spine and that he had osteopenia, as shown by X-rays. This is when I first met John.

John had been admitted to the local hospital for trauma, anemia, a low platelet count, bone pain, and an altered mental status. His blood pressure was elevated, he was obese, his blood sugar was high (consistent with adult onset diabetes), and he felt weak. His total testosterone was very low at 200 ng/dl.

Within 48 hours, John had improved and wished to be discharged. He asked me one question: "How can I get my health back?"

My answer was simple: "You've had an unhealthy lifestyle for 30 years. What you're doing is not working, and you're getting worse, not better. If you're willing to change your diet, exercise, stop smoking, and decrease your alcohol intake, you'll get your health back."

John was lucky because none of his metabolic problems were beyond repair. His high blood pressure and diabetes had not yet damaged his kidneys, and he hadn't had vascular injuries such as heart attack or stroke yet. He had degenerative joint disease, osteopenia, and compression bone fractures. These did not require surgery. His anemia and low platelet count returned to normal levels with hormone replacement therapy and the discontinuation of alcohol.

With the proper knowledge, diet, and exercise, all of his problems could return to normal—and they did. Within six months, he lost body fat, his waist size decreased by three inches, his blood pressure decreased, and his blood sugar returned to normal. His interest in the opposite sex returned when his free and total testosterone blood levels returned to normal. In addition, John's energy level increased, as did his car sales. Even his knee pain lessened. John is now my lifelong friend and patient.

What is Aging?

An aging cell loses the ability to divide, and dies. Cells are genetically programmed to divide a number of times. Cells collectively make up tissues and organs. These tissues and organs function only as well as their component cells. The testes, ovaries, kidneys, and liver lose cell numbers relatively early in the aging body. The muscles, soft tissues, and bones are among the first tissues to show measurable change.

It's difficult to define the aging process as distinct from disease or identifiable pathologic processes that can occur at any age. We do not know exactly what causes aging in every adult, but we've collected a significant amount of data to help explain some of the changes that occur as we age.

In general, distinct muscle changes usually occur in humans in the third decade [8]. We lose 1% of our muscle mass on average every year starting at approximately age 30. Sedentary or inactive non-exercisers lose muscle mass more quickly. Data collected from healthy adults killed in automobile accidents shows significant age-related changes in skeletal muscle area and fiber content. We lose skeletal muscle mass as we age and thus become weaker. Older muscle is also less efficient at protein synthesis than younger muscle of the same size and weight and is thus weaker. This decrease in muscle mass and strength as we age leads to decreased activity. Decreased activity accelerates muscle loss.

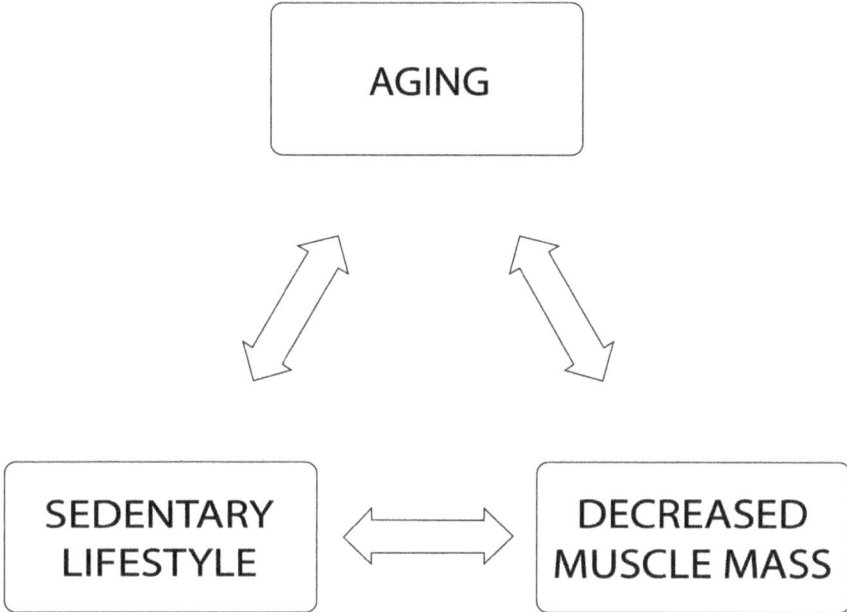

```
                    ┌─────────────────┐
                    │                 │
                    │     AGING       │
                    │                 │
                    └─────────────────┘

         ↗↙                        ↖↘

┌─────────────────┐              ┌─────────────────┐
│                 │              │                 │
│   SEDENTARY     │  ⟺           │   DECREASED     │
│   LIFESTYLE     │              │  MUSCLE MASS    │
└─────────────────┘              └─────────────────┘
```

This age-related change in muscle mass and strength alone leads to a less active lifestyle, continued muscle loss, and a concomitant increase in body fat [9]. It's a vicious, never-ending circle, and it will continue to worsen unless we interrupt the cycle with a change to a healthier life through diet, exercise, increased muscle mass, and hormone replacement therapy as needed.

Body fat measurably increases as we age. Body fat, as described later in this book, produces inflammatory molecules that cause insulin resistance and damage small blood vessels, leading to chronic metabolic diseases and the signs and symptoms of old age. The peak age for body fat mass occurs in adults aged 55 to 71 years [9]. This is not inevitable, but it's totally up to you to do something about it.

```
┌─────────────────────────────────────────┐
│                                           │
│                 AGING                     │
│                                           │
└─────────────────────────────────────────┘
                    ⇓
┌─────────────────────────────────────────┐
│       LOSS OF MUSCLE MASS AND             │
│               STRENGTH                    │
└─────────────────────────────────────────┘
                    ⇓
┌─────────────────────────────────────────┐
│                                           │
│         DECREASE IN ACTIVITY              │
│                                           │
└─────────────────────────────────────────┘
                    ⇓
┌─────────────────────────────────────────┐
│                                           │
│         INCREASE IN BODY FAT              │
│                                           │
└─────────────────────────────────────────┘
```

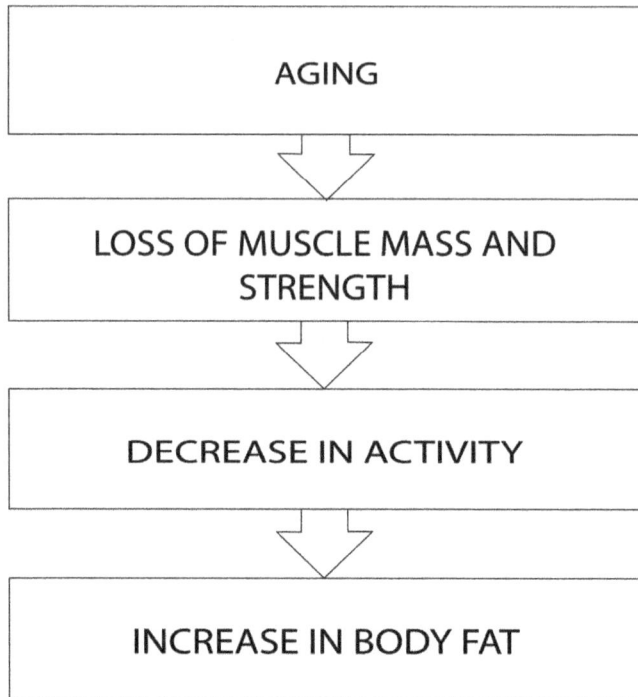

Build Muscle at Any Age

It's possible to change this pattern of muscle loss with nutrition, exercise, and normalizing hormones. Master athletes (defined as performing vigorous exercises four to five times per week) aged 40 to 81 years had similar amounts of muscle mass and strength [10]. Some of the decline in the elderly is due to chronic disuse—lack of exercise.

Nutrition is also very important because protein is required for muscle development. In older muscle cells, higher levels of leucine and essential amino acids are required for muscle growth [11]. **A high-protein diet is essential for muscle growth.**

There is also a decline in sex hormone levels with aging. Men

lose testosterone, and women lose estrogen. **Low hormone levels in both men and women—regardless of cause—increase body fat. These same people show a dramatic increase in muscle mass and loss of body fat when given hormone replacement supplements to return blood hormone levels to median normal values.** Vigorous exercise alone will increase both muscle mass and hormone levels [12]. **Has your doctor checked your hormone levels?**

Both estrogen and testosterone are necessary for muscle growth. Testosterone directly stimulates muscle cell growth. Estrogen stimulates satellite cells, which repair damaged muscle cells and stimulate new muscle growth [13]. Both testosterone and estrogen are needed to maintain and build muscle. Optimal skeletal muscle growth occurs with testosterone levels in the upper levels of normal [15]. It is my firm belief, based on the above studies and data, that it's **possible to build muscle at any age with VIGOROUS EXERCISE, SUPPLEMENTS, A HIGH-PROTEIN/HIGH-FAT DIET, AND MEDIAN NORMAL HORMONE LEVELS.**

Even with the best training and advanced strength and mobility exercises to promote muscle growth at any age, your diet is important. A diet rich in plant and animal essential proteins and essential fats will ensure adequate amino acids essential for muscle growth, muscle recovery and optimal hormone levels. We'll discuss healthy and important fats, essential proteins, and adequate carbohydrates in another section.

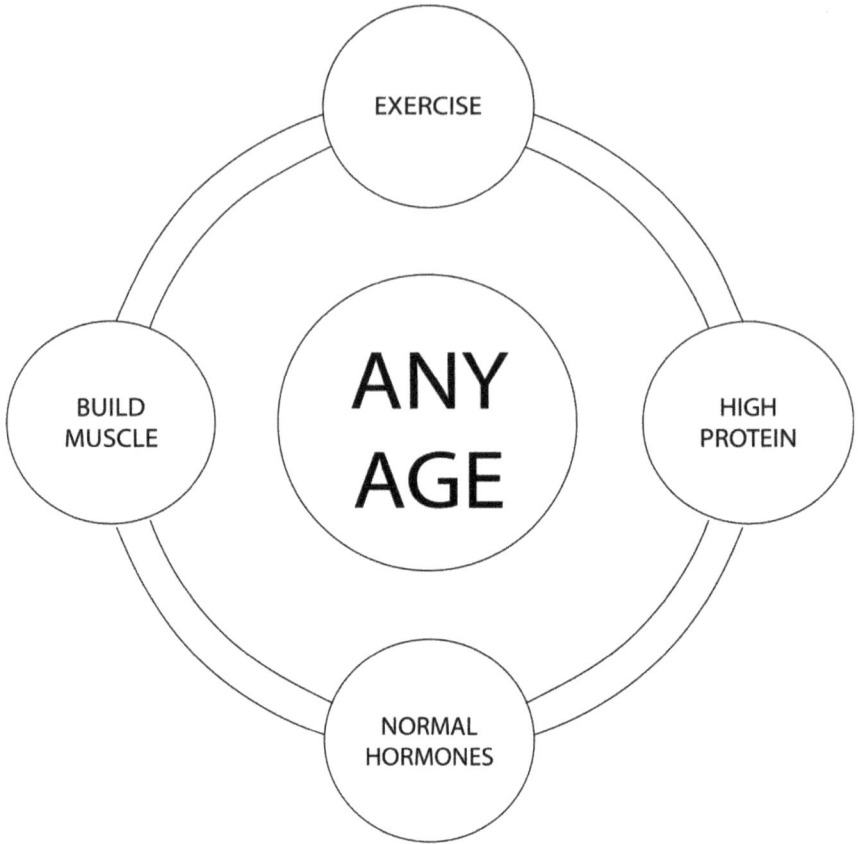

Additional and irrefutable evidence to support this concept are the photographs of bodybuilders in the master age groups of 40 to 80, which are published online after each competition, available at http://musclepapa.smugmug.com.

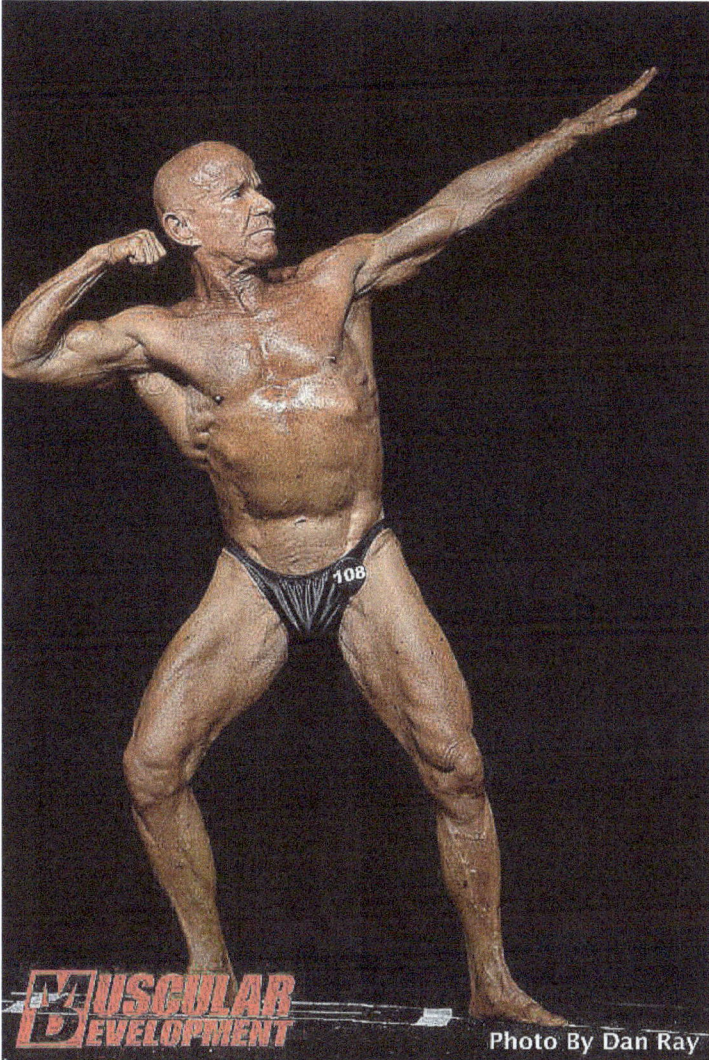

70-Year-Old Athlete

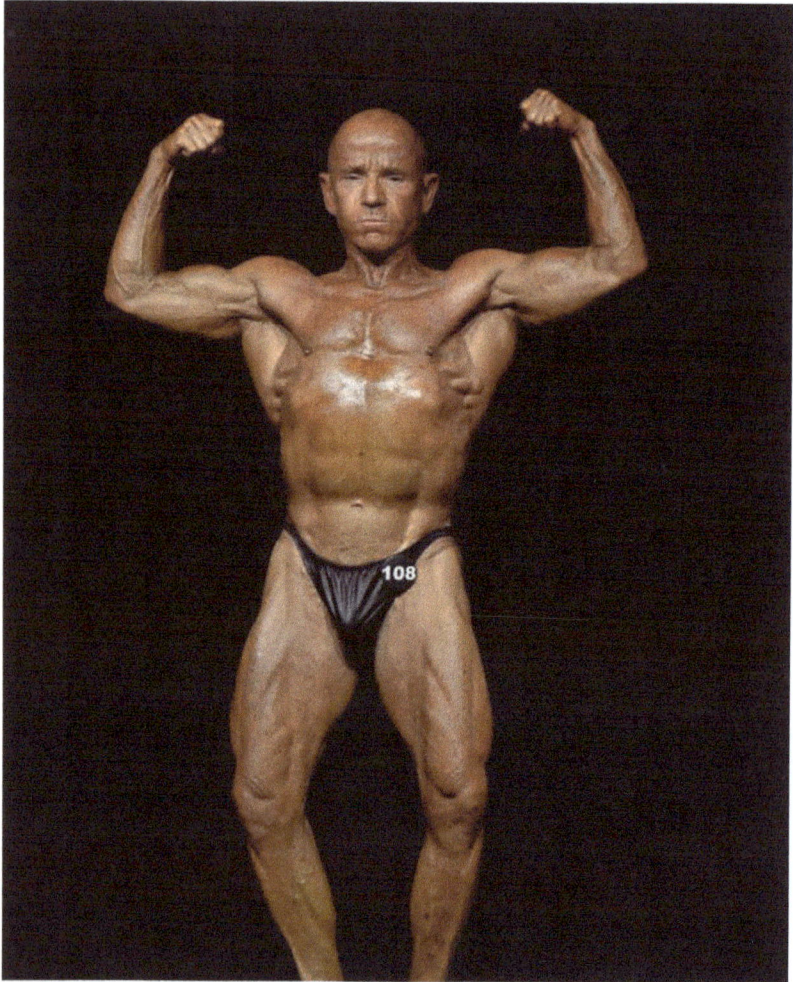

5.7% Body Fat
After 500-Calorie Daily Reduction for
90 Days—Caloric Restriction

Set a Higher Standard for Yourself

From my perspective as a professional trainer of both men and women, my firsthand experience tells me that anyone can get better at any age—*as long as you patiently maintain a healthy lifestyle with diet, exercise, and supplements.*

This is truly the race won by the turtle—one small step in the right direction every day. If you "let go" by smoking, excessive alcohol consumption, and higher caloric food intake, it's not simply the aging process that's making you fat—**it's *you***. If you're in a hurry to lose weight, and choose a crash ultra-low-calorie diet, you'll fail. You'll lose fat, muscle and strength and won't be able to maintain the fat loss. Your brain will automatically lower your metabolic rate and increase your appetite. Your estrogen and testosterone levels will drop, and your cortisol (stress hormone) levels will increase, making you feel weak and depressed [16, 17]. Your new behavior pattern is not sustainable, and you'll return to your previous bad habits. The Minnesota Starvation Study [18] clearly demonstrated that the body attempts to maintain a consistent body weight, and diet alone is not sufficient for you to lose body fat and maintain this loss of body fat. In other words, **DIET ALONE ALWAYS FAILS**. Diet alone fails because your brain set point has not changed, and the brain will not give up. Your brain will lower your metabolic rate and increase your appetite until you gain back the weight you have lost [19].

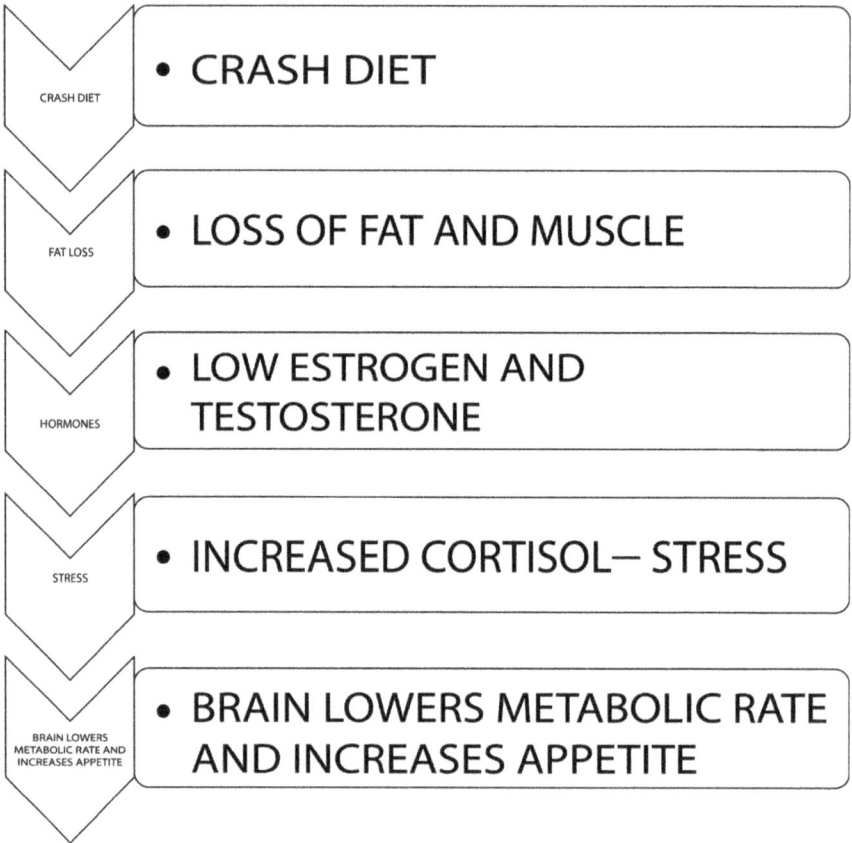

- CRASH DIET

- LOSS OF FAT AND MUSCLE

- LOW ESTROGEN AND TESTOSTERONE

- INCREASED CORTISOL– STRESS

- BRAIN LOWERS METABOLIC RATE AND INCREASES APPETITE

CHAPTER 6
Obesity Defined

Obesity has been defined as an abnormal accumulation of body fat—approximately 20% or more of your ideal body weight. Ideal body weight is the weight for a specific age, gender, and height that has the lowest death rate. How much of your body is bone, muscle, or fat?

Body composition cannot be measured using your height and weight. Obesity by government and insurance standards is defined by a simple formula: body weight multiplied by 703, divided by twice the height in inches. This is your body mass index (BMI). A quick and simple way to determine your BMI is to use your iPad or other tablet and download "BOD keeper" app (bodkeeper.com). This app is very easy to use and is essential, as you'll see later in this book. BMI does not tell you your body composition in terms of muscle mass, bone density and body fat.

A BMI of over 25 by insurance and government standards is considered overweight, and a BMI of 30 or more is obese. Again, this doesn't take body composition into account.

The Centers for Disease Control and Prevention calculates that 69% of adults over age 20 are overweight or obese.

Not every obese person has a metabolic problem, but most do or will develop one. Asians have metabolic problems starting at a BMI of 25; Caucasians at 30; and African-Americans at 35 [19].

In general, obesity is associated with an earlier death [20].

Body fat is divided into two groups: subcutaneous fat (under the skin) and visceral body fat (around and inside organs, such as your liver). It's the visceral body fat that will shorten your life [21].

Subcutaneous body fat is often measured by skinfold calipers. You can purchase a skinfold caliper and measure skinfold thickness in several areas of your body. We prefer the seven-site procedure, which measures the following skinfold sites: abdomen, chest, mid-axilla, subscapularis, supra-iliac, thigh, and triceps.

The numbers are added, and using formulas provided by the caliper manufacturer, your body fat can be calculated. The accuracy, if carefully done, will be within 4% of your true body fat.

This is a good measure to start with for most people, but in reality, you're not measuring visceral body fat. If you're athletic and have less than 10% body fat, this method is not helpful.

Visceral body fat is the dangerous fat that is a proven cause of cardiovascular diseases [22]. A better measure of visceral body fat and cardiovascular risk than BMI is the ratio of your waist in inches divided by your height in inches—your waist-to height ratio or WHtR [23]. This is a very simple measure you can do at home. If your WHtR is less than 50%, you are good. Obesity starts at 57%.

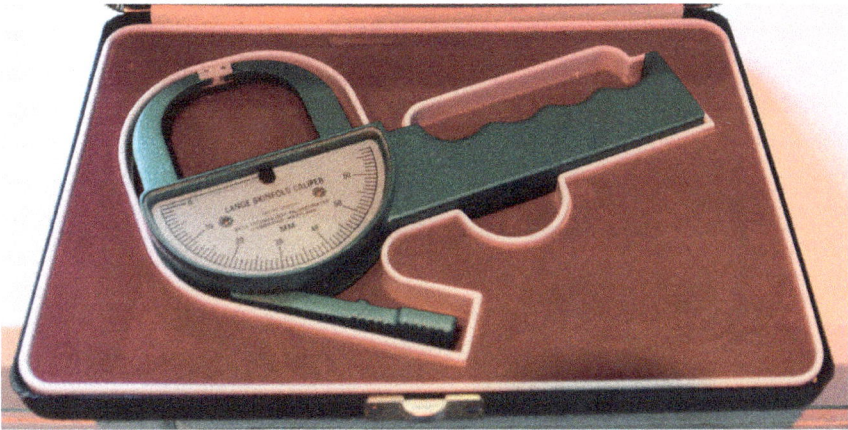

Lange Skinfold Calipers

The next best method of measuring total body fat is by using electrical impedance. A variety of devices are available (from inexpensive to expensive) that measure the resistance of body tissues to an electrical current. This measures total body water, and with this measurement and your weight, a calculation of body fat can be obtained. This technique is dependent upon body water, and your state of hydration will alter the results. This method is a good technique to start with as long as your state of hydration is consistent.

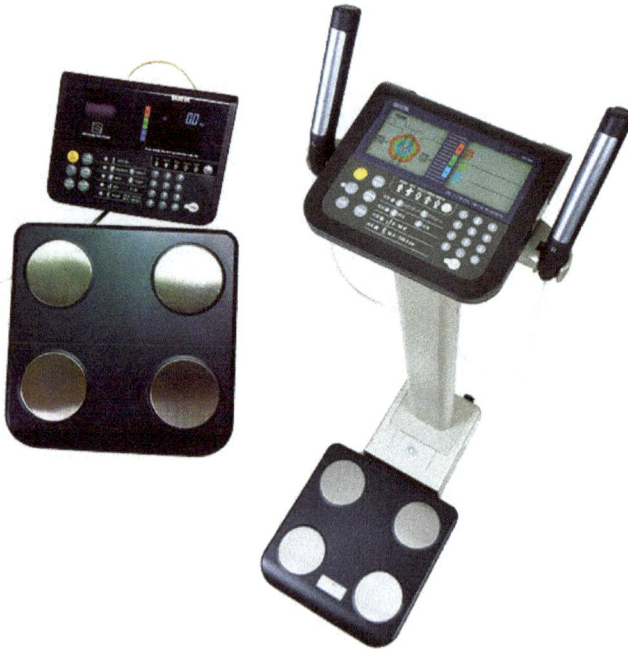

Tanita Electrical Impedance Devices

The most convenient and accurate method of measuring your body fat, muscle mass and bone density is with a DEXA (dual energy X-ray absorptiometry) scan. This is a medical device that uses low-dose X-rays to directly measure body composition. If you're athletic and are serious about body fat reduction, the DEXA scan is your best option since it is accurate and tells you exactly where your fat is located.

I recommend a weekly weight record and a monthly waist-size measurement to start, since these are the least expensive and are very reliable. If you can change your lifestyle for two weeks, these body measurements may give you more incentive to continue your journey to good health.

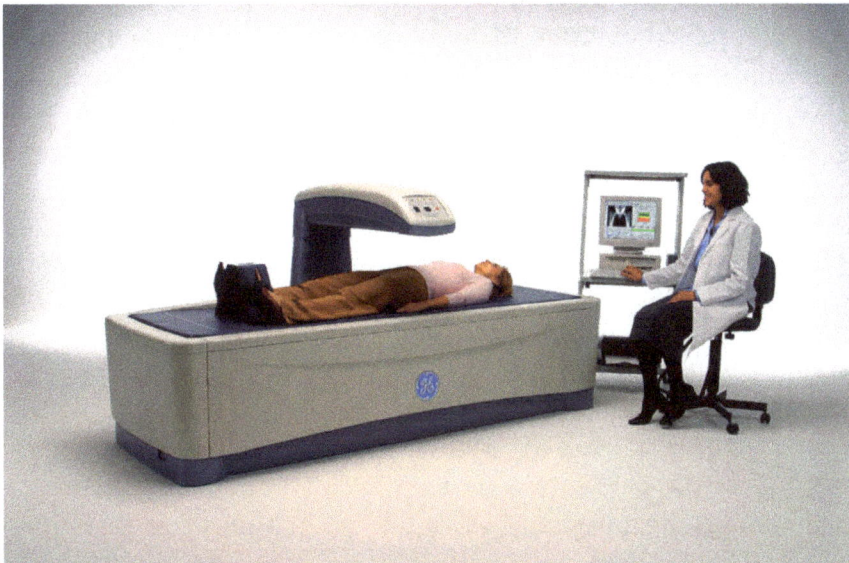

**General Electric DEXA Scanner—
Convenient and Accurate**

Can Surgery Help Obese Patients?

Liposuction reduces subcutaneous fat, and the resulting loose skin can be surgically excised, resulting in a leaner-looking body. However, if an unhealthy lifestyle is the cause of the fat accumulation, surgery will not correct this behavioral problem, and the fat is likely to return over time unless the behavior is changed. Large volume liposuction does not alter a patient's risk for coronary artery disease [24].

Bariatric surgery is currently a surgical treatment for morbid obesity (BMI ≥ 40). Bariatric surgery can be restrictive; restrictive and malabsorptive; reversible; or permanent.

The most frequently performed procedure is a gastric bypass. This is a permanent operation that reduces the size of the stomach and connects this smaller stomach to a portion of the small bowel that bypasses two feet of normal small bowel. This is both restrictive and malabsorptive. Thus, the stomach holds less food, and the reduced size of the small intestine absorbs fewer nutrients.

The lap band procedure is a reversible procedure wherein an adjustable elastic band is placed around the upper portion of the stomach. This decreases the size of the stomach, and less food is able to be eaten.

Both procedures result in weight loss. Gastric bypass can improve insulin-resistant diabetes, but long-term studies show that these benefits will disappear in 24% of patients within three years [25]. The reason for the loss of benefit is that these patients have not embraced a healthy lifestyle.

Complications of gastric bypass include diarrhea, Vitamin B12 deficiency, iron deficiency, ulcers, secondary hyperparathyroidism, and pain. In one-year, three-year, and five-year post-bariatric surgery follow-ups, weight loss was found to be 76.8%, 69.7% and 56.1%. Thus, weight gain occurs in a significant proportion of patients over time [26]. In addition, there is a high incidence of alcohol abuse post bariatric surgery [27].

It's difficult to treat a behavioral problem with surgery; an unhealthy lifestyle is the underlying problem, and this is not surgically correctable.

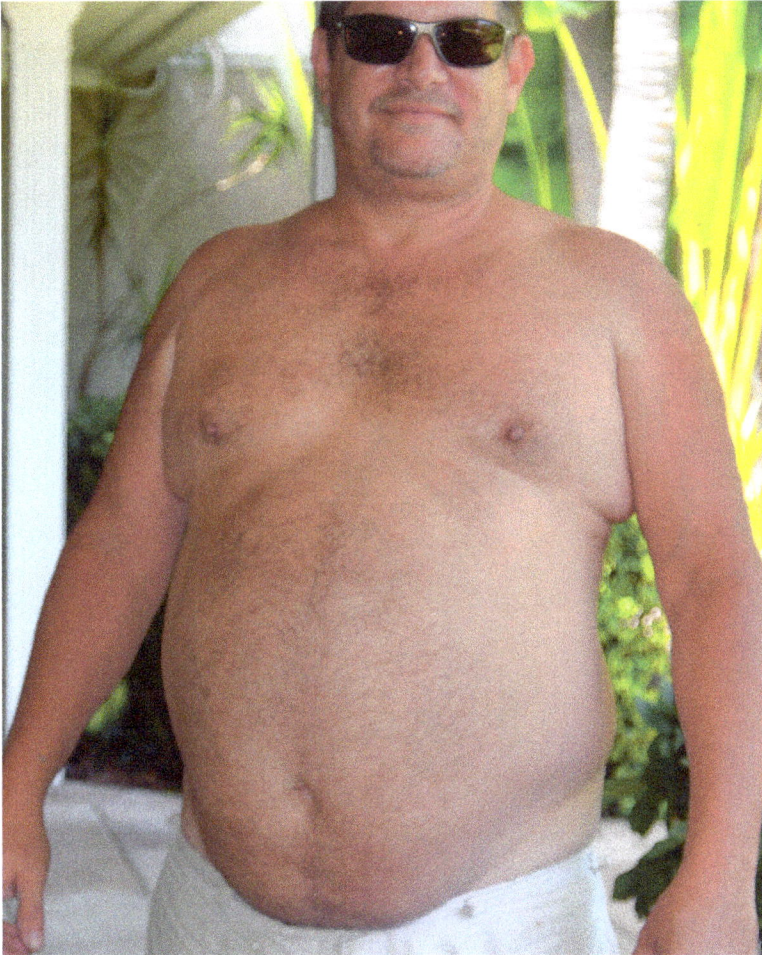

Visceral Body Fat—Is This You?

CHAPTER 7
How Your Body Works—
Let's Start at the Beginning

Diet—What You Eat

The most important part of your healthy diet is your knowledge of food and of how your body uses food to create body fat and muscle and prevent disease. Most of us learn about food from our parents, and we all assume that we know what's healthy to eat. Because most people have no idea of which foods are healthy, insulin-resistant diabetes, heart disease and obesity are major health problems. Do fat parents have fat children? The answer to this is unequivocally yes [1]. Do most parents recognize this? No. What's missing is knowledge.

There is no diet that fits all people equally. Your food choices are part of a healthy lifestyle that achieves your goals and continues over your entire life. Your diet is a pathway to a lifetime of health. Your diet should not be a race to lose weight—but if it were a race, it's a race won by the turtle and not the hare. Think of your diet as one small daily step toward your goals. **The most important thing regarding a healthy life is calorie restriction [3].** Many experts say, "Do not count calories." This advice is not optimal, because at some point in your new lifestyle, your body will change—you will plateau or stop losing body fat. This requires a change in your

43

diet to continue on your healthy path. To correct this plateau, you will need to know what exactly you are eating. **If you can measure something, you can control it. Calorie counting is a tool to help you change your diet when your diet no longer works. All diets are trial and error, since no two people are alike.** Weighing your proteins is a good method to keep track of the fat and protein that you are eating. Carbohydrates are more difficult to control if you do not count calories.

Digestion

Food can be classified as proteins, carbohydrates, fats, fiber, and micronutrients (vitamins and minerals). You put food in your mouth. You chew your food into smaller bits and swallow, and the mix enters your stomach.

Once in the stomach, hydrochloric acid (HCl) continues the process of breaking the food into smaller bits. HCl is very important because it breaks down proteins into amino acids, activates other digestive enzymes, and prevents bacterial overgrowth. Both stomach HCl production and digestive enzyme production decrease after age 65 [2]. This decrease may cause indigestion and heartburn. Thus, not all stomach problems are caused by *increased* stomach acid, and antacid medication is *not* universally helpful.

The mix of food then enters the small intestine, where the digestive process is completed. Enzymes digest proteins into amino acids, fats into fatty acids, and carbohydrates into simple sugars (glucose and fructose). Fiber in the mix slows the rate of absorption of these nutrients; fiber itself is not digested.

The mix of amino acids, sugars, and fatty acids then goes directly to the liver via the hepatic portal vein for immediate use and also enters the bloodstream. **The pancreas detects these three classes** of nutrients (macronutrients) in the blood and releases insulin to remove these nutrients. Insulin converts sugars into fat and liver glycogen; amino acids are assembled into muscle cells; and fat is converted to fatty acids, which are stored in fat cells as triglycerides.

What is a Calorie?

[A calorie is a unit of measure that has been applied to all food groups. A calorie has been defined as the amount of heat required to raise one gram of water by one degree centigrade. Thus, the relative energy value of all foods can be measured in a science lab. Your body, however, does not metabolize all food groups in the same manner, and calorie content is not the best measure of food value. It's more important to know how your body uses each type of food macronutrient (fat, protein and carbohydrates).]

Calories are useful to find a starting point for your diet and a general plan for each type of food. The bottom line in a healthy diet is that you achieve your goals and you do not develop the chronic metabolic diseases that decrease your quality of life and longevity. Calorie restriction is the one indisputable path to longevity [3]. **This means that at the end of each week, CALORIES COUNT.**

The Actions of Insulin

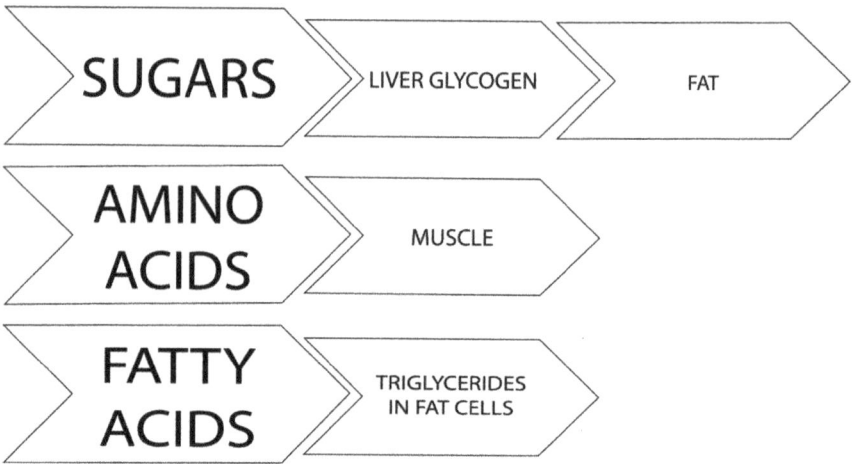

SUGARS	LIVER GLYCOGEN	FAT

AMINO ACIDS	MUSCLE

FATTY ACIDS	TRIGLYCERIDES IN FAT CELLS

Fat in the Diet is Essential

Fat in the diet is essential. You must have fat in your diet.

Fat is a source of energy for cells, containing 9 calories per gram as compared to the 4 calories per gram that both carbohydrates and protein contain. **Yet it is not the fat in your diet that makes your body fat.**

Fat is a component of every cell membrane and is thus necessary for healthy tissues. It's a component of nerve cells and is essential for nerve conduction and brain function. All steroid hormone synthesis (testosterone and estrogen) is based on the cholesterol molecule, and cholesterol is an essential fat. **The most recent data suggests there is no link between saturated fat consumption and heart disease, diabetes, or obesity [3].**

There is one group of dietary fats that are unhealthy without controversy—trans fats. Trans fats are usually man-made saturated fats produced by hydrogenating vegetable oils. These trans fats do not spoil quickly, and so they produce products that have longer commercial shelf lives. Trans fats have been used to make margarine and packaged baked goods such as cookies, crackers, and snack cakes. All man-made trans fats have been proven to increase the risk of cardiovascular disease, and the U.S. Food and Drug Administration (FDA) is in the process of eliminating trans fats from the food supply. Always check product labels on your packaged foods for trans fats. If the label uses the word *hydrogenated*, there are trans fats in the food, and you should not eat this food.

Body Fat and Sugar—How You Become Fat

The more sugar in the blood, the higher the insulin levels and thus the greater production of fat. When insulin levels are low, triglycerides residing inside fat cells get broken down into fatty acids for energy, and the fat cells shrink in size—this is a decrease in body fat.

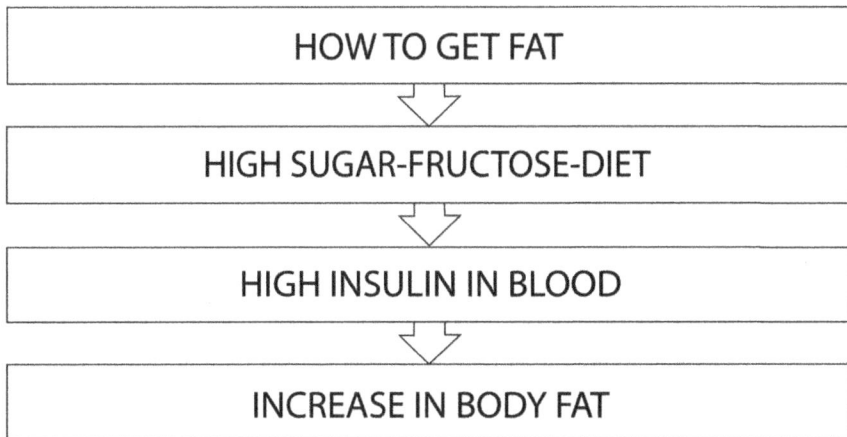

HOW TO GET FAT

HIGH SUGAR-FRUCTOSE-DIET

HIGH INSULIN IN BLOOD

INCREASE IN BODY FAT

Hormones control the speed that these metabolic processes occur—from the hypothalamic portion of the brain, from the pituitary gland, and from the thyroid gland [5].

Leptin is a hormone produced by fat cells. Leptin helps the body regulate energy balance by inhibiting the sensation of hunger. When leptin is released into the bloodstream, it tells the brain that you have enough energy stored as fat, and to reduce your appetite. Low leptin levels tell the brain that food intake is low, and so the brain slows the body's rate of energy consumption (metabolic rate). The body tries to maintain a steady state (homeostasis), and when fat is high, leptin is high, and the metabolic rate increases to compensate for the increased energy available. When fat is low, leptin decreases and again the brain keeps the body constant by decreasing the metabolic rate.

Serum leptin levels correlate with body fat levels and can be used as a measure of your body fat.

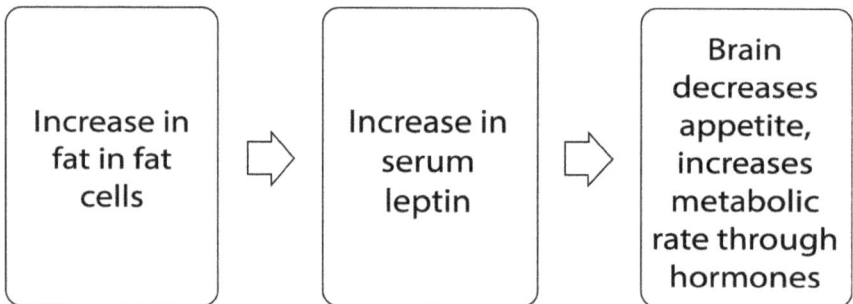

| Increase in fat in fat cells | ⇨ | Increase in serum leptin | ⇨ | Brain decreases appetite, increases metabolic rate through hormones |

How Your Body Works

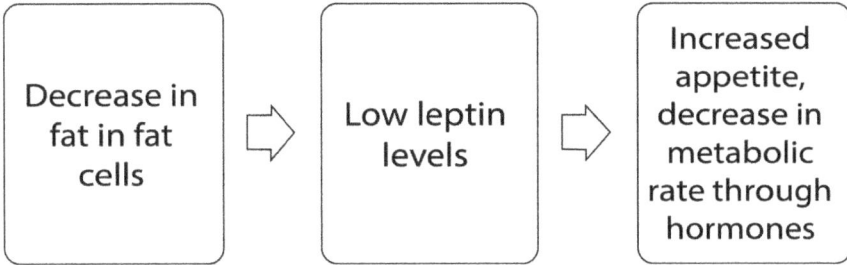

Decrease in fat in fat cells	⇨	Low leptin levels	⇨	Increased appetite, decrease in metabolic rate through hormones

Your body muscles and organs require a source of energy while the fat cells store and save energy. High insulin levels direct macronutrients into storage, while low insulin levels direct nutrients into direct use for energy. **A new finding reveals that high insulin levels can block leptin function and cause both a low metabolic rate and simultaneous fat storage.** The presence of high insulin levels is the real problem, since insulin creates body fat. With high insulin levels, the leptin signal causes no decrease in appetite, and energy expenditures do not increase. **This is how we become obese and morbidly obese.**

How Not to Become Fat

It is possible to change this. Here are a few simple steps to take:

1. Decrease insulin production by eliminating foods with high sugar content and low fiber content, such as juice, cakes, pies, candy, milk products, soft drinks, bread, and pasta.

2. Consume protein/fat foods with each meal to increase satiety and increase metabolic rate.

3. Increase intake of foods with fiber, such as all vegetables and salads, to slow the absorption of all nutrients.

4. Increase exercise and increase the number and quality of the mitochondria inside your muscle cells, building more muscle cells and thus increasing your metabolic rate. More muscles equals more calories burned while you rest.

5. Stress reduction and adequate sleep will lower insulin levels by decreasing cortisol production.

In summary, high insulin levels determine whether we become fat by blocking leptin and by creating body fat. The number and size of fat cells determine your body fat. You make fat cells during the first two years of life, and this is determined by factors beyond your control. **However, the *contents* of these fat cells is under *your* control and is determined by insulin; the more insulin you make, the more fat is stored in your fat cells.**

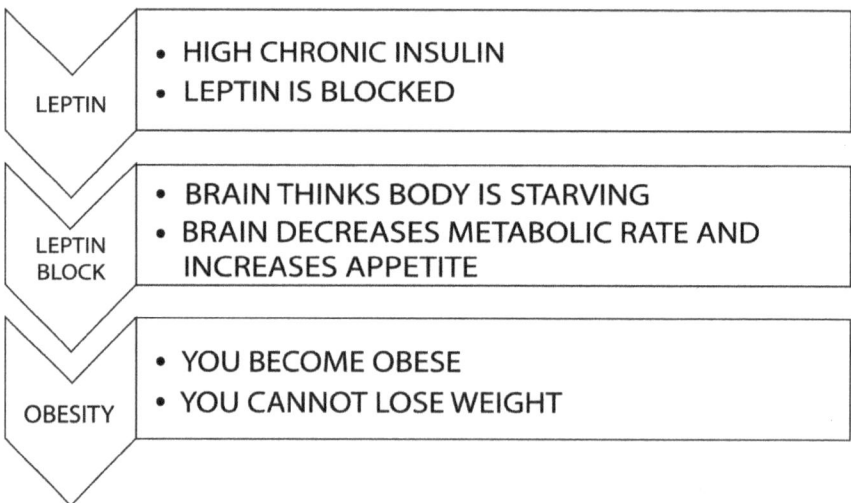

LEPTIN
- HIGH CHRONIC INSULIN
- LEPTIN IS BLOCKED

LEPTIN BLOCK
- BRAIN THINKS BODY IS STARVING
- BRAIN DECREASES METABOLIC RATE AND INCREASES APPETITE

OBESITY
- YOU BECOME OBESE
- YOU CANNOT LOSE WEIGHT

It is very important to decrease insulin levels and your total body fat by way of a diet low in sugars and a lifestyle that burns sugars and builds muscle through exercise. Sugar is needed if you wish to build muscle, and this requires some degree of intelligent carbohydrate cycling, which will be discussed later in this book.

We need some fat as a healthy source of energy, but modern lifestyles and certain foods lead to disease. Let's return to the digested food in the small intestine. Carbohydrates are broken down into glucose and then released into the bloodstream.

The liver now converts some of this glucose into glycogen (a healthy form of energy storage in the liver). Fat in the small intestine is converted into fatty acids. Fatty acids are processed by the liver and linked to lipoproteins so they can be transported to all the cells in the body and then used as an energy source or be stored in fat cells.

Protein in the diet is converted into amino acids in the small intestine and is used to build and maintain muscle cells. Any excess is converted into fat by the liver as well, but this process consumes as much energy as it produces. Thus, the liver must deal with the excesses in our diet.

When glycogen storage in the liver is full, this fat must be stored outside the liver in fat cells, the majority of which are located in your abdomen as visceral body fat. Some of this fat is also stored under your skin as subcutaneous body fat. Thus, excessive caloric intake *does* count and *does* lead to a fat body.

Stress and Bad Behavior

Stress is a physiological and biochemical event that occurs when your brain perceives a threat. Stress ultimately causes the release of cortisol by the adrenal glands. Other hormones may be released as well, including norepinephrine, epinephrine, testosterone, and estrogen. Stress begins in the brain and affects the entire body. The elevated cortisol levels cause an increase in appetite by increasing activity in the parasympathetic nervous system and the vagus nerve. Cortisol increases blood pressure and blood glucose and thus increases insulin release and body fat.

We all experience stress, and some people experience more stress than others. When stress is transient, the cortisol level returns to normal, and all is well. Prolonged stress is harmful. It is chronic or prolonged stress that really creates problems. Prolonged elevated cortisol levels raise blood glucose and, subsequently, insulin levels. Eventually, the body's cells stop responding to the constantly elevated insulin—this is known as insulin resistance. Insulin resistance causes type 2 adult onset diabetes and a variety of metabolic problems.

Stress also causes insomnia, and the brain interprets this as an additional stress and so causes even more cortisol to be produced. With chronic cortisol overproduction, blood sugar increases, as do insulin levels. The insulin blocks the effect of leptin on the brain, and the brain sees only low leptin levels and so increases appetite [6].

Again, a high insulin level produces fat, and low leptin function decreases the metabolic rate, and so we get fatter.

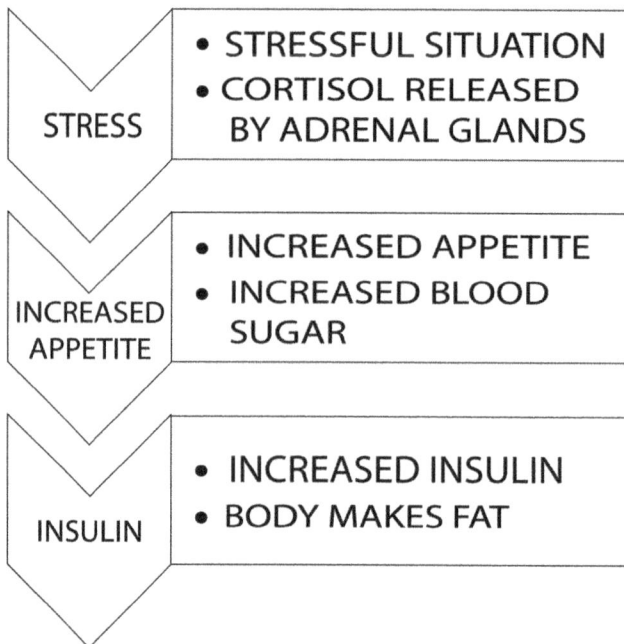

STRESS
- STRESSFUL SITUATION
- CORTISOL RELEASED BY ADRENAL GLANDS

INCREASED APPETITE
- INCREASED APPETITE
- INCREASED BLOOD SUGAR

INSULIN
- INCREASED INSULIN
- BODY MAKES FAT

Big Mike's Story

Big Mike is a patient of mine with chronic high insulin levels. Mike is morbidly obese with a large, protruding belly (high visceral body fat). Early in life, he developed bad eating habits. Eating food became his way of reducing stress. Whenever life became difficult, Mike would eat something sweet to provide immediate stress relief and pleasure. This pattern of behavior became his pattern of life-sugar addiction. This fixation with food was a severe psychological problem with inevitable results. He would chronically overeat, drinking a gallon of whole milk and enjoying high-calorie desserts every day. He enjoyed a sedentary lifestyle, and at an early age, he developed insulin-resistant diabetes.

His pancreas initially produced high insulin levels, and his body cells became resistant to insulin. Eventually, his pancreas stopped producing insulin, and to prevent low blood sugar, his doctor placed him on injectable insulin. This is called type 2 or maturity onset diabetes. This returned his blood sugar to a more normal level and also allowed Mike to continue overeating.

Eventually, his belly became so large that he had to change the position of his back and hips in order to walk upright. This alteration in his gait led to severe lower back and neck pain, as well as severe degenerative joint disease. Today, Mike is unable to walk. He continues to overeat and self-medicate with insulin and remains morbidly obese. He is essentially homebound despite being under 70 years of age.

If you find yourself using food for emotional stress relief on a regular basis, here are some suggestions:

1. Don't purchase or possess any of the foods that you usually use for stress reduction or pleasure.

2. Plan and prepare all your meals in advance, and eat each meal at a defined or specific time.

3. Find a different activity for stress relief. The best and most effective stress-relieving activity is exercise. Other stress-relieving activities include computer use, reading books, massage, shopping, meditation, yoga, and Pilates. None of these activities will make you obese.

Why Body Fat is Bad

As your body ages, it's the excess body fat that increases the risk of hypertension, insulin-resistant diabetes, coronary artery disease, stroke, dementia, and bone and joint injury [7, 8].

Fatty tissue makes up a large percentage of the cells in your body. Men average between 18% and 24% body fat; women average 25–31% body fat. Fat cells can become dysfunctional and accelerate age-related diseases, while one's life span is extended by caloric restriction and a reduction in visceral fat [9]. Fat cells store energy—fatty acids in the form of triglycerides. Fatty tissue is located beneath the skin (subcutaneous) and around vital organs (visceral). Visceral fatty tissue is the largest endocrine organ in your body. **Visceral fat produces hormones and cytokines that affect body temperature, metabolism, immune function, wound healing, and sex.** It is theorized that with increased fat cell replication, fat cell precursors become dysfunctional with age, and in the presence of chronic high insulin levels, produce inflammatory products (tumor necrosis factors) that damage blood vessels and other tissues, causing the pathologies associated with obesity and aging [10, 11].

Statistics from the NIH reveal a 14-year reduction in life expectancy in extremely obese adults. The reason fat people die younger can be attributed to the production of inflammatory molecules by the fat cells that injure small blood vessels in the heart, kidneys, brain, and liver. This cell damage results in metabolic syndromes—the chronic metabolic diseases discussed already.

Is Dietary Fat Bad?

Many scientists have tried to prove that dietary saturated fat is unhealthy [12, 13]. This area has been controversial in the past, but multiple recent studies clearly show that dietary **saturated fats do not raise the risk of heart disease** [14].

A meta-analysis (a statistical technique for combining the results from multiple studies) of 21 studies encompassing 350,000 subjects for more than 20 years showed no association of saturated fats with coronary heart disease [15, 16].

Many experts recommend decreasing dietary saturated fats to raise HDL, and lower LDL by changing to plant-based diets ("Level IV data"—see the chapter on supplements.) Remember, it is the small particle LDL that causes vascular damage. **Saturated fats do raise total cholesterol by increasing HDL and the harmless large particle LDL. The small particle LDL is harmful and is not increased by eating saturated fat. Sugar raises small particle LDL.** We will discuss this in detail in the paragraphs on plant-based diets. This also means that studies using total cholesterol or total LDL as endpoints are not valid. In the meantime, keep eating.

In the past, many studies replaced fat calories with carbohydrate calories, but this did *not* decrease the incidence of coronary artery disease. In this discussion, you need to keep in mind that the liver will convert all excess protein and carbohydrates to fat for storage—calories *do* count, and caloric restriction has always worked to prolong longevity.

The Ugly Fat

Trans fats increased the risk of coronary artery disease as found in the Nurses' Health Study and are thus considered to be harmful. Trans fats raise LDL, lower HDL, and increase C-reactive protein—an additional marker for coronary artery disease. These trans fats are fats created by heating vegetable oils in the presence of hydrogen gas. Trans fats have longer shelf lives and are ideal for frying fast foods. In June 2015, the FDA decided to ban all man-made trans fats from the food supply. Measures of total cholesterol alone are of little value.

The Nurses' Health Studies, started in 1976 by Dr. Frank Speizer and in 1989 by Dr. Walter Willett, are long-term studies of the health of female nurses. The studies followed 121,700 female registered nurses since 1976 and 116,000 female nurses since 1989 to assess risk factors for cancer and cardiovascular disease.

CHAPTER 8
Ligands, Insulin Resistance and Metabolic Syndrome— Why Insulin Resistance is Bad

All biologic systems depend upon the ability of cells to communicate. Cells communicate by using messages called ligands. Ligands are molecules that bind to other molecules to create a new effect. Ligands released into the circulation seek out specific cells by looking for specific receptors on cell surfaces. The desired communication between cells occurs when a cell surface membrane receptor and a chemical ligand come together. The result of the binding of a ligand to a cell receptor is a new activity or new protein in the cell.

How Your Cells Communicate

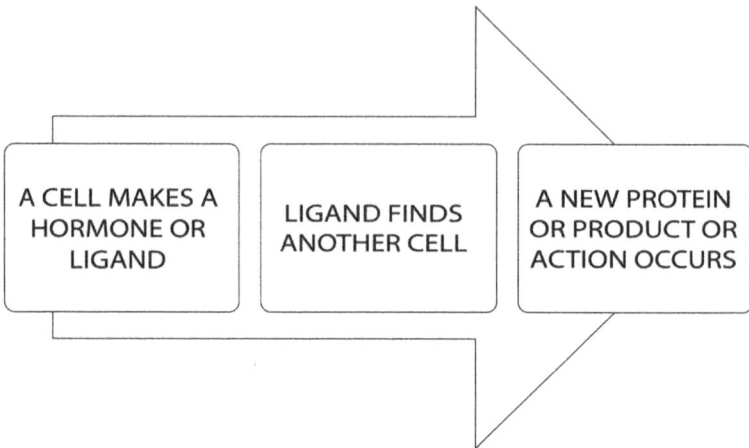

A CELL MAKES A HORMONE OR LIGAND	LIGAND FINDS ANOTHER CELL	A NEW PROTEIN OR PRODUCT OR ACTION OCCURS

The cell receptors are metabolically active and can increase in number as more ligands are presented. It is also possible that in the presence of excess ligands, the receptor activity can decrease or become resistant. This is the theoretical reason why human cells become resistant to excess insulin. The results of this are known—insulin resistance results in higher blood sugar levels. The pancreas detects this increase in sugar and produces more insulin, making things even worse. Eventually, the cells of the pancreas fail because they are overworked, and diabetes results. The liver then decreases the storage of sugar by decreasing the production of glycogen from glucose. Insulin-resistant fat cells no longer take up circulating lipids, and this increases the fatty acids in circulation, leading to elevated serum triglycerides. Fat cells lose the ability to store triglycerides. These abnormal lipids in the bloodstream—specifically small, low-density lipoproteins (LDL)—stick to and damage the walls of arteries, thus producing arterial disease throughout the body.

Insulin resistance is associated with the presence of increased blood pressure (hypertension). Approximately 50% of people with hypertension are insulin-resistant [1].

[In non-insulin-resistant people, insulin causes dilatation of blood vessels. In insulin-resistant people, no dilatation occurs due to the failure of cells in the blood vessel linings to release nitric oxide. The smooth muscle cells surrounding the blood vessels restrict blood flow, causing a compensatory increase in pressure. Blood flow is ultimately decreased [2, 3]. This is also how we develop hypertension, erectile dysfunction in men, peripheral vascular disease, and coronary artery disease. Poor blood flow to the penis or vagina affects a person's ability to become aroused and have sexual intercourse.]

Nitric oxide in pill form can be increased to palliate these conditions, such as in nitroglycerin pills, sildenafil (Viagra, Cialis etc.), and a variety of over-the-counter supplements.

Metabolic Syndrome and Organ Damage Caused by Chronic Insulin Overproduction

1. High blood pressure (hypertension)

2. High blood sugar (type 2 or adult onset diabetes)

3. Abnormal lipids (hyperlipidemia)—elevated LDL

4. Coronary artery disease (heart disease)

5. Peripheral vascular disease

6. Stroke (brain damage)

7. Kidney damage

It is important to remember that the only lipid particle proven to damage small blood vessels is the small particle LDL. The large particle LDL is relatively harmless.

```
┌─────────────────────────────────────────────────────────────┐
│                    CHRONIC HIGH INSULIN                       │
└─────────────────────────────────────────────────────────────┘
                             ⇓
┌─────────────────────────────────────────────────────────────┐
│           INSULIN RESISTANCE AND PANCREATIC FAILURE           │
└─────────────────────────────────────────────────────────────┘
                             ⇓
┌─────────────────────────────────────────────────────────────┐
│                  LIVER STRESS AND DYSFUNCTION                 │
└─────────────────────────────────────────────────────────────┘
                             ⇓
┌─────────────────────────────────────────────────────────────┐
│  ELEVATED SERUM GLUCOSE, TRIGLYCERIDES AND SMALL-DENSITY LIPOPROTEINS  │
└─────────────────────────────────────────────────────────────┘
                             ⇓
┌─────────────────────────────────────────────────────────────┐
│                    DAMAGED ARTERY WALLS                       │
└─────────────────────────────────────────────────────────────┘
                             ⇓
┌─────────────────────────────────────────────────────────────┐
│                   DIABETES, HYPERTENSION                      │
└─────────────────────────────────────────────────────────────┘
                             ⇓
┌─────────────────────────────────────────────────────────────┐
│                       HEART DISEASE                           │
└─────────────────────────────────────────────────────────────┘
```

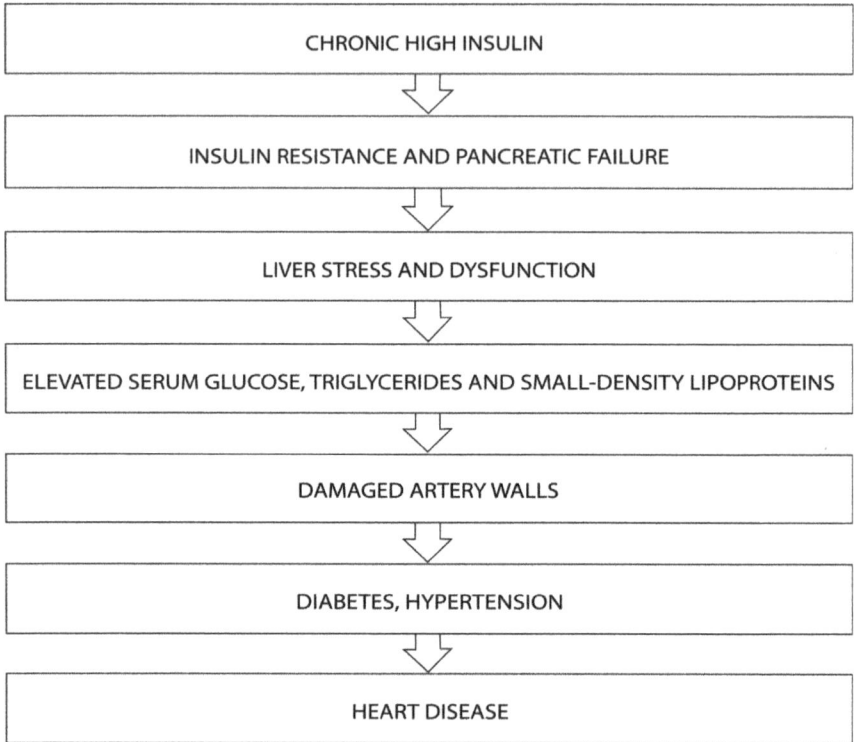

The metabolic syndrome is a group of medical conditions defined by the presence of any three of these conditions: high blood sugar, high triglycerides, low high-density lipoproteins (HDL), visceral obesity, and hypertension. Approximately 34% of Americans have a metabolic disease [4].

Metabolic syndrome is a precursor leading to diabetes, heart disease, and death. You won't die from obesity, but you will eventually die from its resultant metabolic syndromes.

Carbohydrates Are Complicated

Carbohydrates are the sugars that are the usual source of energy for your cells. Plants produce carbohydrates. The sugar in your blood is glucose. Your food contains many different forms of carbohydrates: fructose is the sugar in fruit; galactose is the sugar in milk; table sugar or sucrose contains one unit of glucose and one unit of fructose; starch contains many units of glucose (polysaccharide); fiber is comprised of carbohydrates that are not digested.

Carbohydrates are digested in the stomach and small intestine into sugars (glucose and fructose). When glucose enters the bloodstream, insulin is secreted by the pancreas, and glucose then enters all of the body's living cells, where it's immediately used as an energy source. Glucose can be stored in the liver as glycogen for future use. Excess glucose not burned for energy, nor stored as glycogen in the liver or muscles, is converted to triglycerides and stored in fat cells.

The liver can store between 80-100 grams of glycogen, and the muscles in the body can store 300-600 grams of glycogen (depending on total body muscle mass).

Fructose occurs in fruit and is always combined with glucose. Fructose is more harmful than glucose because it can only be metabolized by liver cells. Fructose in excess is not converted to benign glycogen but is converted to fatty acids, triglycerides, and harmful low-density lipoproteins [5]. This leads to insulin resistance, and, thus, **your 12-ounce glass of orange juice in the morning is just as unhealthy as 12 ounces of Coca-Cola.** (Actually, the Coke has less fructose and may prove to be healthier.) Alcohol (ethanol) is even worse since it can cause direct cell damage to the brain and heart, in addition to requiring liver-only metabolism, as does fructose.

The ability of a carbohydrate to enter the bloodstream as glucose

can be measured relative to pure glucose, and this is called the **glycemic index.** A high-glycemic-index food, such as white bread, elevates your blood glucose level faster and much higher than does a low-glycemic carbohydrate, such as broccoli. Fiber is an important aspect of glycemic index, since high fiber reduces the glycemic load of foods by delaying absorption of food in the small intestine.

Fiber is a plant product (carbohydrate) that humans cannot digest. It is beneficial in slowing the absorption rate of nutrients (sugars and fats). This slower rate of glucose absorption lowers peak insulin levels and helps to maintain lower insulin levels. The slower the absorption of fructose, the lower the amount of metabolic stress on the liver. The delayed fat absorption moves fat into the colon, where it can be eliminated. **Sugars are used by cells for energy or are stored as fat, but they are never eliminated. You either burn sugar or you wear it.**

The fiber in food makes it healthier because the sugar is more slowly absorbed, and peak insulin levels are lower. Eat the whole food, but don't blend it or make a smoothie because all you are doing is decreasing the effective fiber content and increasing peak insulin levels.

An additional source of fiber frequently overlooked is flax meal. Flax meal is made from finely ground flax seeds and provides fiber and omega-3 fatty acids. We recommend two tablespoons of flax meal daily. **There are no essential carbohydrates.** Your body can use fat as a source of energy when carbohydrates are not available.

Protein

Protein is present in the inner and outer portion of every cell. Cells make up your tissues. Your body can store carbohydrates in the form of fat, but not protein. The protein in your food (poultry, fish, beef, dairy, and some plants) is broken down into amino acids in the stomach and small intestine. These amino acids are then reassembled into the tissues of your body relatively quickly. Your body is in constant repair and in constant renewal of tissues and needs amino acids to do this work. Protein is essential. Approximately 20% to 30% of your calories should come from protein.

According to Dr. Jonas Frisen, **your body (with the exception of the brain) renews itself completely every 7 to 10 years.** The liver converts excess amino acids into glucose or fat. Exercise causes muscle growth and muscle repair and increases the need for protein in the diet. Exercise in the absence of sufficient amino acids can cause tissue damage. If you exercise, you need to eat enough protein to maintain or improve your muscles.

C-Reactive Protein

C-reactive protein (CRP) is made by the liver in response to ligands or products produced by white blood cells (macrophages) and fat cells. CRP is a measure of the amount of inflammation present in your body. **This is usually in the presence of dying or injured cells,** and CRP activates the innate immune system (a complementary system) found in the liver to help the body remove dead cells. CRP elevations can occur with exposure to environmental toxins and diets rich in heavy metals and trans fat.

CRP decreases with any long-term increase in exercise. Exercise reduces the incidence of coronary artery disease, and this decrease in CRP may be part of the reason exercise is beneficial [6].

Dietary Fat

Approximately 30–40% of your dietary calories should come from the fat in your diet. Dietary fat is an important source of fuel for the cells of the body, providing 9 calories per gram of fat, while carbohydrates and proteins provide only 4 calories per gram. Fats are a very important part of your diet.

The fat-soluble vitamins (A, D, E and K) are essential dietary nutrients found in the liver and fatty tissues of animals. Fats (glycerophospholipids) are the main structural component of all biologic cell membranes. All steroid hormones, including cortisol, estrogen and testosterone, are made from fats—lipids.

All the fat in your food is comprised of combinations of fatty acids that differ in the number of hydrogen atoms attached to the carbon atoms. A saturated fat, such as butter, has more hydrogen atoms than does a monounsaturated fat, such as olive oil. Unsaturated fats are found in plants, vegetable oils, seeds, fish and nuts. Saturated fats are the fats found in animal meat, dairy products, coconut products and palm products.

The digestion of fat in the small intestine is complex and requires the presence of lipase, bile salts, phospholipids, and transport lipoproteins. The dietary fat is broken down into triglycerides and fatty acids. Fatty acids can be stored in fat cells and can be used as a source of energy. Once inside the small intestine, the fatty acids, cholesterol and fat-soluble vitamins form chylomicrons that allow fat to enter the lymphatic circulation and subsequently the large veins of the chest and then into the liver. (Chylomicrons are lipoprotein particles consisting of triglycerides (85–92%), phospholipids (6–12%), cholesterol (1–3%), and proteins (1–2%). They transport dietary lipids from the intestines to other locations in the body.)

Unsaturated Fats

OLIVE AND NUT OILS

NUTS: ALMONDS, WALNUTS, PECANS

AVOCADOS AND SEEDS

FISH

Saturated Fats

ANIMAL MEAT: BEEF, CHICKEN, PORK

MILK PRODUCTS, CHEESE

COCONUT AND PALM PRODUCTS

Fat—Measured by Blood Tests

Fat is not water-soluble and cannot circulate in the bloodstream unless it's converted into a lipoprotein complex by the liver. These lipoprotein complexes are measured by blood tests called lipid profiles.

Fats processed and released as carriers of lipids, called apolipoproteins, are classified according to their density. Very low-density lipoproteins (VLDL) carry newly synthesized triglycerides from the liver to fat cells for energy storage. Low-density lipoproteins (LDL) carry phospholipids, cholesterol, and triglycerides throughout the body to cells for repair and for energy. High-density lipoproteins (HDL) transport phospholipids, cholesterol, and triglycerides from the cells of the body back to the liver.

The size of LDL particles varies from large and buoyant to small and dense. Small, dense LDL is especially rich in cholesterol and is associated with atherosclerotic heart disease and other diseases of vascular damage. The increased pathology of small, dense LDL derives from less-efficient hepatic LDL receptor binding, leading to prolonged circulation and exposure to endothelium and increased oxidation.

Apolipoprotein synthesis in the liver is controlled by many factors: dietary composition, alcohol, fructose, hormones, vitamins and drugs. When stressed by dietary excesses, such as alcohol, trans fats, high insulin levels, and medications, the liver's apolipoproteins can cause disease. The stressed liver produces C-reactive protein, which is a measure of inflammation and is a risk factor for diabetes, insulin resistance, and coronary artery disease [6].

The low-density small particle (LDL) is directly associated with coronary artery disease.

Increased Risk of Coronary Artery Disease

HIGH SMALL-PARTICLE LDL

LOW HDL

HIGH C-REACTIVE PROTEIN

When Does Your Body Make Fat?

Your body makes fat whenever your body makes insulin. Thus, whenever you eat a meal, your blood glucose increases, and your pancreas produces insulin to return your blood glucose level to normal. This is when your body makes fat.

Conversely, **when you're asleep, you're fasting, and your body may consume body fat as a source of energy.**

The Value of Antioxidants

It is logical to expect that antioxidants would be beneficial, since they eliminate the free radicals or reactive oxygen species (ROS) that damage DNA and cause cell death. We are under constant attack from free radicals. They're in the air and the sunlight that hits our skin. **Free radicals are produced whenever a cell generates energy from food.** Free radicals steal electrons from other molecules and can damage cells and change metabolic processes.

Our bodies have developed molecules that donate electrons in order to neutralize free radicals, and these are antioxidants. There are many types of antioxidants, and each is unique and acts in a specific situation. Our bodies are continuously using them. Vitamin C, Vitamin E, and Coenzyme Q10 are some examples. There are hundreds more. Antioxidants are now being marketed just like fast food—all good, all the time. Yet the antioxidants already present in our fruits and vegetables are sufficient to protect us from cell damage, and there is little evidence that increasing our intake through supplements is beneficial.

The antioxidant beta-carotene, when taken as a pill/supplement, actually increases the risk of lung cancer in smokers. [7]. There is one exception, and that is in the prevention of the eye disease called macular degeneration, where an antioxidant mixture of beta-carotene, Vitamin E, Vitamin C, and zinc is beneficial [8].

Reactive Oxygen Species and Mitochondria

[Reactive oxygen species (ROS) are chemically reactive molecules containing oxygen (one example is peroxide). ROS are involved in many biologic events occurring in both health and disease. Mitochondria are independent parts of the insides of cells, and they use oxygen and glucose to produce energy in the form of adenosine triphosphate (ATP).

Mitochondria are the engines inside cells, and ATP is the fuel for the cell. Mitochondria can divide when stimulated by energy demands, such as by exercise or work. There are discrete changes in the mitochondria of aging cells that contribute to the dysfunction seen in aging cells, especially the skeletal muscle cells. Mitochondria produce ROS as a signal to the cells that oxygen is limited, and the ROS induce responses to save the cells. In this situation, ROS are good.

Older mitochondria may become dysfunctional and produce excess ROS, which causes problems and predisposes one to metabolic syndromes. ROS are produced by the activated cells of the cellular immune system (when antigenic peptides are presented to T-lymphocytes). T-cells or T-lymphocytes are a type of lymphocyte that plays a central role in cell-mediated immunity. A peptide antigen triggers the immune system to develop antibodies to that peptide. Peptides are short strings of amino acids. Longer chains are known as proteins.

ROS are then produced as part of the inflammatory response. Skeletal muscle produces ROS during contraction in hypoxic (low oxygen) conditions. Excess ROS can damage skeletal muscle and are implicated in the loss of muscle cells in immobilized muscle and underutilized muscle. ROS are implicated in age-related diseases and cancer.

To combat the overproduction of ROS, cells produce antioxidants such as thioredoxin and glutathione [9].]

In diabetes and obesity, there is a chronic excess of extracellular glucose and fatty acids producing excess ROS, causing insulin resistance and lipid deposition in the liver, heart, and pancreas. ROS have a role in insulin resistance [10].

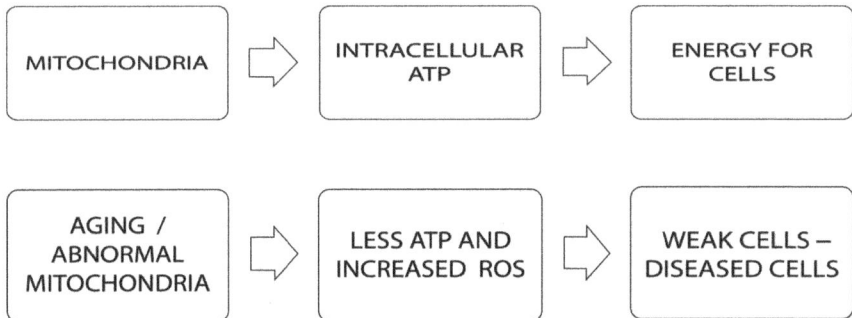

MITOCHONDRIA ⟹ INTRACELLULAR ATP ⟹ ENERGY FOR CELLS

AGING / ABNORMAL MITOCHONDRIA ⟹ LESS ATP AND INCREASED ROS ⟹ WEAK CELLS – DISEASED CELLS

CHAPTER 9
Diet

How to Eat

The next question is, How and what to eat? The answer depends on your goals. There's a difference between sports that require the participants to perform an action (such as gymnastics) and sports that are purely aesthetic (such as bodybuilding). There's also a difference between endurance sports (such as marathon running), speed sports (such as speed skating), and strength sports (such as weightlifting). Some wish to build muscle, lose body fat, increase energy level, and/or appear physically younger. The two most important principals are: you must know what's healthy for you to eat, and you must be in control of what you eat.

In order to be in control of what you eat, you must measure it. If you measure it, you can control it. I recommend an accurate scale and a daily written or electronic journal. The journal should contain a daily or weekly record of your weight, waist size, exercise activity, and quantitative food choices. Trial and error are expected. As your body changes, so must your diet.

Body weight does not distinguish between muscle weight and fat weight. Measuring your waist size can be helpful as a measure of visceral body fat. Most people don't have regular access to the more accurate methods of measuring body fat, such as DEXA scans or Bod Pods (a machine that measures body mass when you sit inside of it).

The use of electrical impedance can be helpful, but only the expensive equipment is accurate. Simple skin calipers that measure skin thickness (subcutaneous fat) can be helpful but don't measure visceral body fat.

I recommend taking a simple photograph of your body every four weeks with your mobile phone, and use the BOD Keeper app. The photo should be dated and kept with your other records. Using your computer, iPad or other tablet, or mobile phone for your record keeping is best. This will help to measure your progress and provide motivation to continue along your path.

According to research conducted by Fitbit, seeing an unflattering photographic image is a powerful source of motivation for losing weight. It certainly was for me!

The *best diet* is controversial, and the important aspect of food choice is that it achieves your goals and keeps you on a healthy path for life—one small step at a time. You need to ask yourself each week, "Am I better today than I was last week?" The answer should be, "Yes, I'm better—and I can prove it." Your journal will provide a behavior pattern that will help you to be successful in achieving your goals.

There should be no time pressure. Your path is comprised of small steps in the right direction. You've likely been bad for 20 or more years, and this can't be corrected in just weeks or months. Remember, this is a race won by the turtle.

The number of meals one should eat per day depends on your work requirements, lifestyle, and it is a controversial subject. There is no *best number of meals.*

My recommended dietary preferences are based on science, tradition, and common sense. The science is that of the Paleolithic diet, which includes food choices of our early ancestors and excludes most milk products, most grains, and processed foods [1]. Followers of this Paleolithic diet since childhood do not get obese nor get diabetes, hypertension, coronary artery disease, or stroke [2].

The non-scientific, traditional aspect of my diet mimics the diet recommended for bodybuilders, since my goal is to build muscle and decrease body fat. Not all aspects of the traditional bodybuilding diet have been scientifically tested, but the results are visible at competitions.

The common sense part of the diet is, if it works, continue; if it doesn't work, change something."

If you'd like, you can skip the scientific part of this discussion and go straight to the list of healthy foods and the quick diet method.

Calories Count, and You Need Fat in Your Diet

In order to lose weight, you must change the type of food you are eating. Fat, protein, and carbohydrates have different effects on your body. **In general, a weight-loss diet means you will be consuming fewer calories.** Fat increases your metabolic rate and is an essential nutrient, while carbohydrates are not essential. With regard to simple weight loss—simple means loss of fat, bone density and muscle—macronutrients don't matter. It doesn't matter whether it's high or low-carbohydrate, high or low-protein, or high or low-fat; as long as the total calories are lower, you will lose weight.

Macronutrients—protein, carbohydrates, and fat—are very important in determining which tissues you lose—muscle, fat or bone—as well as what energy level you will have. A simple low-calorie diet alone is not a healthy diet because you will lose bone density, muscle mass, as well as body fat, and your brain will increase your appetite and lower your metabolic rate.

Intelligent Caloric Restriction

One important fact [#1] that must be carved in stone is that in every species, including primates (human beings, apes and monkeys) caloric restriction increases longevity [4, 5]. This is the most important fact regarding your diet. One theory to explain this phenomenon is that with fewer calories but sufficient essential minerals, amino acids, and vitamins (thus, no malnutrition), there is less oxidative stress on the mitochondria in muscle cells [6]. Mitochondria are small structures inside all living human cells that produce energy for cells. The analogy is that mitochondria are like the batteries that run the cell. Less oxidative stress means less damage to the DNA in the cell's mitochondria, leading to healthier muscle cells. To date, why calorie restriction prolongs lifespan is not fully known. A more recent scientific explanation of the benefit of calorie restriction (CR) is the Informational Theory of Aging proposed by Dr. David Sinclair in his book *Lifespan*. In this theory, the stress of calorie restriction activates the longevity genes that force cells to divide less and reuse spare parts to maintain energy and prolong cell life. This important process is called autophagy, and we will return to this subject in chapter 19.

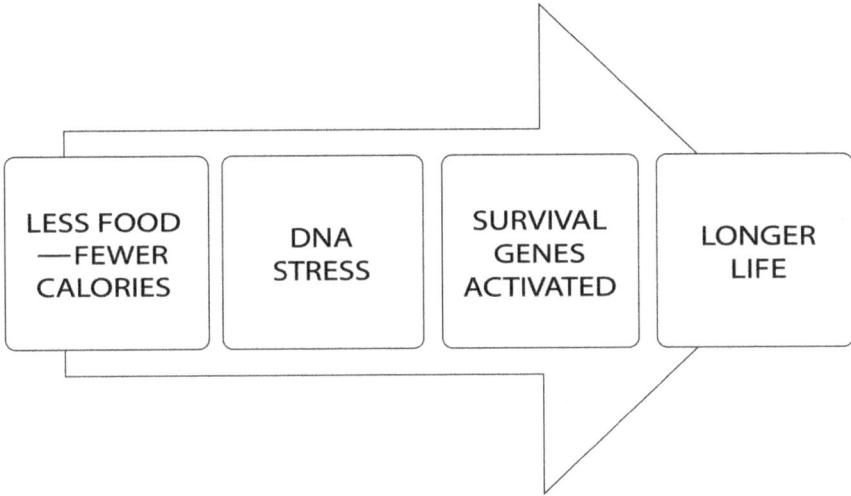

LESS FOOD —FEWER CALORIES → DNA STRESS → SURVIVAL GENES ACTIVATED → LONGER LIFE

FACT NUMBER TWO—we have only three variables that we can control with regard to our health: diet/food, activity/exercise, and supplements/medicines/hormones.

According to the American Diabetes Association report of June 2014, 29.3 million Americans, or 9.3% of the U.S. population, have diabetes. In seniors over 65 years of age, 25.9% were diabetic. Medical complications of diabetes include high blood pressure, abnormal lipids, heart disease, stroke, blindness, kidney disease, and amputations. The total cost of diabetes to U.S. taxpayers in 2012 was approximately $245 billion. Much of this could have been saved by lifestyle changes, including diet, exercise, supplements and hormones.

It's not just a problem in the U.S. either. According to the World Health Organization in 2014, the global incidence of diabetes in adults over 18 years of age was 9%.

Fasting and Ketosis

Fasting is a behavior during which no calories are ingested. It may cause a state of ketosis, where stored fats are broken down for energy, resulting in a build-up of acids called ketones within the body if prolonged. Fasting is part of many religious practices, and it has some beneficial effects. The Ramadan fast is intermittent, occurring only from sunrise to sunset, and ketosis does not usually occur, nor is there any change in aerobic or cardiovascular athletic performance [7].

The ketogenic diet and ketosis were first studied scientifically by Vilhjalmur Stefansson and Eugene F. DuBois at Bellevue Hospital as a possible medical treatment [8]. There is evidence that a ketogenic diet will help epilepsy, obesity, and diabetes.

If you eat few carbohydrates—fewer than 20 grams/day—your glucose reserves become depleted after two to three days [9]. Ketone bodies are produced by the liver in this low-glucose environment to maintain energy levels. Ketone bodies are a source of energy when glucose is not available. Ketone bodies produce more energy than does glucose due to greater mitochondrial ATP (adenosine triphosphate) production. Protein in the diet limits the use of amino acids as a glucose source and increases satiety. Body fat decreases, owing to increased lipid oxidation and decreased body fat production. In muscle cells, mTOR (mechanistic target of rapamycin) is an enzyme that regulates cell growth and division in response to energy levels, growth signals, and nutrients. This mTOR signaling is decreased during ketosis, and this limits muscle growth [10]. This means that on a ketogenic diet you cannot build new muscle. Recent studies in humans showed that five days of fasting each month, for three consecutive months, reduces body weight, trunk, and total body fat; lowers blood pressure; and decreases insulin-like growth factor 1 [27].

In summary, a very low-carbohydrate diet will help you lose body fat, *but* you will not be able to build muscle. You may experience greater fatigue initially. It's possible for your body to function normally as well.

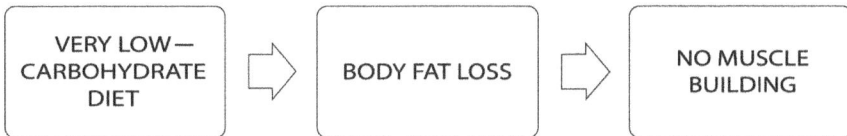

```
┌─────────────────┐      ┌─────────────────┐      ┌─────────────────┐
│   VERY LOW—      │      │                 │      │   NO MUSCLE     │
│  CARBOHYDRATE    │  ⇨   │  BODY FAT LOSS  │  ⇨   │   BUILDING      │
│      DIET        │      │                 │      │                 │
└─────────────────┘      └─────────────────┘      └─────────────────┘
```

How Many Meals Per Day is Best?

Bodybuilders and many other athletes and dieters frequently eat a small meal every three to four hours. The thinking is that smaller meals increase the metabolic rate, lower insulin peaks, reduce hunger and lessen the risk of going off the diet. However, in controlled feeding studies, there was no significant difference between three meals per day and more than three meals per day [11]. Fewer than three meals per day did result in an increase in perceived appetite and hunger, along with less appetite control. DO NOT SKIP A MEAL. Eat at least 3-4 meals a day to prevent loss of appetite control.

Resting Energy Expenditure (REE)
Feel Free to Skip This Section and go to the Quick Diet

My diet starts at an arbitrary point based on resting energy expenditure (REE), with the expectation that this starting point will change. Remember that every diet requires trial and error and change. The units of the diet are calories, and this is for convenience.

We will calculate a total daily calorie intake based on REE and modify this based on activity level [12]. For simplicity, you may skip this diet and go to the easier Quick Diet.

Men:

10 x Weight(kg) + 6.25 x Height(cm) – 5 x Age(years) + 5.

Women:

10 x Weight(kg) + 6.25 x Height(cm) – 5 x Age(years) – 161.

Please visit www.calorieline.com/tools/tdee. This site will calculate your REE for you.

We now modify this number by multiplying activity level:

No exercise = REE x 1.2

Active 3 days/week = REE x 1.375

Very active 3 days/week = REE x 1.55

Very active 5 days/week = REE x 1.725

Very active 7 days/week = REE x 1.9

A 40-year-old male, height 5'10", weighing 160 pounds, who is active three to five days per week, will need 2,545 calories per day to maintain his weight, and 2,045 calories per day to lose one pound per week. This is a precise number to be used as a **starting point** only. This number will change as your body changes. Trial, error, and re-evaluation are key elements to achieve your goals. Keep a written record.

We are not ready to eat just yet, since we still need to determine the proportions of the macronutrients—protein, carbohydrates, and fat. This is another discrete value and will need modification in time if it does not work and as your body changes. Since our presumed goal is building muscle and losing body fat, we will need approximately

30-40% of our calories as proteins, 20-30% carbohydrates, and 30-40% fats.

If you're pear-shaped (thick endomorph), you will need 40% protein, 20% carbohydrates, and 40% fats. If you're muscular athletic (meso-morph), you will need 40% protein, 30% carbohydrates, and 30% fats. If you're thin and lean (ectomorph), you'll need 35% protein, 25% carbohydrates, and 40% fats.

I suggest starting with 35% protein, 30% carbohydrates, and 35% fats for convenience only.

Now, with a calorie goal and macronutrient proportions, we can pick food groups.

- ***Daily Protein:***
  2,045 calories x 35% = 716 calories.
  4 calories per gram of protein.
  716 / 4 = 179 grams of protein per day.

- ***Daily Carbohydrates:***
  2,045 calories x 30% = 613 calories.
  4 calories per gram of carbohydrates.
  715 / 4 = 153 grams of carbohydrates per day.

- ***Daily Fat:***
  2,045 calories x 35% = 716 calories.
  9 calories per gram of fat.
  716 / 9 = 80 grams of fat per day.

Thus, a 40-year-old male, height 5'10", weighing 160 pounds, who is active three to five days/week, will need 2,045 calories per day to lose one pound per week and build muscle, and he will eat 179 grams of protein, 153 grams of carbohydrate, and 80 grams of fat every day.

How many meals per day is optimal to build muscle and lose body fat? This has been discussed, and three or more meals per day will work. The important points: eat when you're hungry; never skip a meal, since you won't be able to control your appetite; stop eating when nearly full—never overeat; always include a protein source in your meals to maintain satiety and to build muscle; and avoid eating for four hours prior to bedtime. However, if you awaken early and are hungry, please do eat, since you don't want muscle cells to be used as your energy source. Sleep is essential to decreasing cortisol levels and maintaining adequate leptin levels.

I suggest four to five meals per day in order to maintain a high-protein diet. Drink two liters of liquid per day, or enough liquid to keep your urine colorless.

Here are five sample meals containing approximately 500 calories per meal ("p/c/f/cal." = protein, carbohydrates, fat, calories):

- *½ cup of old-fashioned oatmeal made with water*
  p/c/f/cal. = 5/27/3/150

- *5 eggs*
  p/c/f/cal. = 31/0.6/20/370

- *½ cup blueberries*
  p/c/f/cal. = 0.5/10/0.25/40

- *3.5 oz. salmon*
  p/c/f/cal. = 40/0/7.6/240

- *2 whole-wheat pita*
  p/c/f/cal. = 8/48/2/240
  salad as desired—all you wish

---

6 oz. skinless chicken breast
p/c/f/cal. = 52/0/6/280

200 grams peeled yam
p/c/f/cal. = 3/48/0.2/206
Salad as desired—all you wish

---

5 oz. broiled sirloin steak
p/c/f/cal. = 43/0/10/285

200 grams baked potato with skin
p/c/f/cal. = 4.6/51/0.2/210
salad as desired

---

8 oz. codfish
p/c/f/cal. = 50/0/2/218

195 grams long-grain brown rice
p/c/f/cal. = 5/45/1.7/216
Salad as desired

Now, please forget the above data collection and go down to my Quick Diet below. Please keep your own electronic or paper food diary and measure your results. If you're losing inches from your waist or one pound per week, you're doing well and should continue eating healthy food without all the precise measurements.

If all goes well, you should eat anything you desire one day a week. Yes; one day of no restrictions! During this free day, healthy carbohydrates will increase your leptin levels and increase your metabolic rate (REE) since your body has been losing fat. Fat loss tends to lower leptin levels and REE. In order to maintain REE while building muscle and losing body fat, you must have an intense exercise program that raises your hormone levels. Supplements also become important.

Yes, we're attempting to change your body. You can lose body fat and build muscles at any age.

The Quick Diet

A simple method to help create a diet plan is to go to the Mayo Clinic calorie calculator (www.mayoclinic.org/calorie-calculator/itt-20084939) to calculate your daily calorie needs. This is your resting energy expenditure (REE)—the number of calories your body uses every day.

Now subtract 500 calories from this number to determine your one-pound-loss-per-week daily diet calories. Since our goal is to build muscle, we need 1-1.5 grams of protein per pound of body weight. Since protein in nature is always accompanied by fat, you'll have sufficient fat as well. Thus, weigh your protein and calculate the calories using the MyFitnessPal app or website. Subtract the protein calories from your diet calories, and the remaining calories are available for carbohydrates. This quick diet assumes that you will exercise. Green vegetables and salads may be eaten without restraint since the calories to metabolize them are equivalent to their calorie content, and the fiber is important. The MyFitnessPal.com website (not the mobile app) is excellent for finding the macronutrient and calorie content of most foods.

The Quick Formula for Protein, Fat and Carbohydrates in Your Diet

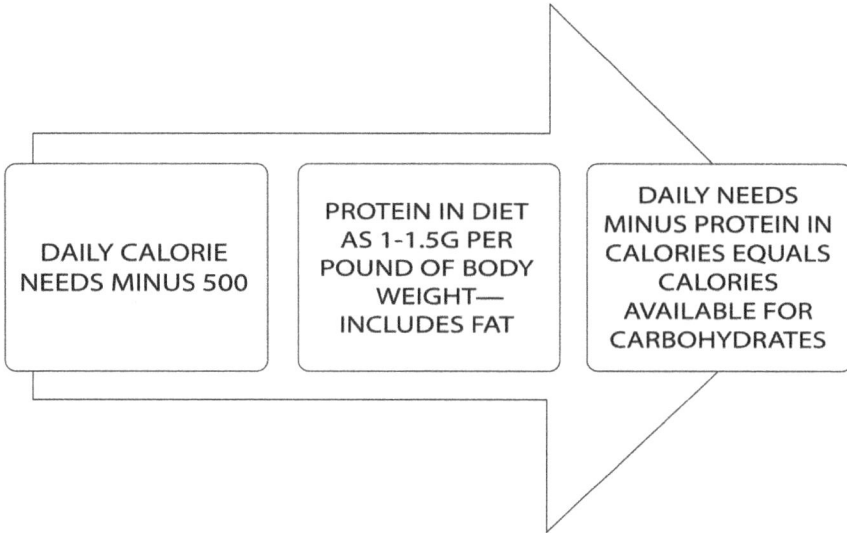

DAILY CALORIE NEEDS MINUS 500	PROTEIN IN DIET AS 1-1.5G PER POUND OF BODY WEIGHT— INCLUDES FAT	DAILY NEEDS MINUS PROTEIN IN CALORIES EQUALS CALORIES AVAILABLE FOR CARBOHYDRATES

Quick Diet Formula—Example

(Mayo Clinic Calories – 500) minus (calorie content of 1.5 x body weight in pounds of protein choices) = calories available for carbohydrates. Thus, a 40-year-old male, weight 160 pounds, who is active three to five days per week, will need 2,045 calories per day to lose one pound per week and build muscle (179 grams of protein per day). (Six large 2-ounce eggs = 36 grams of protein and 426 calories; 6 ounces of Atlantic wild salmon = 38 grams of protein and 348 calories; 8 ounces of chicken breast = 50 grams of protein and 240 calories; 8 ounces of lean steak = 48 grams of protein and 400 calories.)

The above four protein meals total approximately 172 grams of protein and 1,414 total protein and fat calories. This leaves 2,045 – 1,414 = 631 calories remaining for carbohydrates.

This is a good place to start. Protein shakes made from whey protein and low in carbohydrates can be substituted for a meal. Remember, as long as you're moving in the direction of your goals, you're doing well. If you plateau—and you will!—you just need to change something. The only things *you* control are your food choices, your exercise program, and your supplements/medicines and hormones.

In my personal diet, when preparing for a bodybuilding competition, I always plateau at some point. When I plateau, I just eliminate anything that will block leptin—gluten, MSG, and artificial sweeteners. Since insulin is the major leptin blocker, I increase my fiber with salads and limit my intermediate/high-glycemic carbohydrates to small servings of oatmeal, yams, and rice. If this doesn't work, then I limit my protein sources to fish and chicken (both dark and white meat) and decrease or eliminate my protein shakes. I also eat more green vegetables and salads and decrease the rice and yams. The fat content is important to remain constant.

This diet isn't a specific diet for all readers but rather outlines a simple method of finding a starting point for anyone's diet when knowing only calorie count and protein requirements.

We All Need to be Athletes: Protein From Food

We've discussed the essential role of protein in your body. To summarize, protein is essential to build and repair your tissues. Athletes need a high-protein diet [13]. For us to remain healthy, we need to exercise and be athletes, and try to eat 1 gram of protein per pound of body weight. Bodybuilders need up to 3.6 grams per pound, and possibly more [14]. Fat is also very important, and there are no essential carbohydrates.

Healthy foods include whole eggs, fish, shellfish, chicken, turkey, lean beef, lean lamb, lean pork loin, and unflavored Greek yogurt. Protein is also available from vegetable sources such as legumes, broccoli, peas, nuts, and spinach. Animal sources of protein are best. There is a measurable decrease in total testosterone production in athletes eating a vegetable protein diet compared to athletes who eat proteins from animal sources. This decrease occurred after just six weeks [15].

Protein Supplements

Protein supplements are powders or premixed powders made from milk, eggs, or plants. The most popular protein supplement is whey protein made from milk. Whey protein is rapidly absorbed. If lactose intolerance is a concern, lactose-free whey protein is also available in the form of whey isolate or whey hydrolysate.

Casein protein is also made from milk and is more slowly absorbed than whey. Egg protein is absorbed even more slowly. Egg and whey protein supplements are equal in their ability to stimulate muscle growth in animals [16].

Soy protein is controversial. The Harvard School of Public Health, as of February 2014, gives soy protein mixed reviews—their "Straight Talk" is not so straight. The concerns regarding the estrogen-like isoflavones in soy protein is still a topic of research. Much depends upon the amount of soy protein in your diet and how your gastrointestinal bacteria help to metabolize isoflavones [17]. Other noncontroversial plant-based protein supplements are available, with pea proteins being a good source.

Fat in Your Food: The Media, Politics, and Bad Science of Heart Disease— Who Controls Cultural Knowledge?

The most tragic story regarding health during the last 65 years is the high incidence of coronary artery disease in the U.S. Doctors today expect patients, as they age, to have some coronary artery disease and high blood pressure. Your heart is mostly muscle tissue that works continuously. Coronary artery disease occurs when the coronary arteries that supply your heart muscles accumulate fatty plaques that impede blood flow to the muscle. When blood flow stops, the muscle area involved dies, and this is called a heart attack, or myocardial infarction. When your heart muscles are starved for blood, you get chest pain called angina. When your weakened heart muscles cannot pump blood out of the heart, you become short of breath and can go into congestive heart failure.

According to the Centers for Disease Control and Prevention, 610,000 people die of heart disease in the U.S. every year—that's one in every four deaths [18].

Heart disease is the leading cause of death for both men and women. More than half of deaths due to heart disease in 2009 were in men. Coronary heart disease is the most common type of heart disease, killing over 370,000 people annually. Every year, about 735,000 Americans have a heart attack. Of these, 525,000 are a first heart attack, and 210,000 happen in people who have already had a heart attack [19]

Some of the blame for these deaths can be attributed to bad science, politics, and the media. Public opinion and public behavior can be the measures of our cultural knowledge, and from the 1950s to the present, our cultural knowledge blamed cholesterol, red meat, and saturated fat in the diet for causing the increase in heart disease. This thinking was inaccurate, and only recently has the truth emerged that the blame belongs on trans fats and carbohydrates—especially sugar.

The incorrect thinking was as follows: fat in the diet causes fat to accumulate in the arteries that supply the muscles of the heart. The arteries get clogged—much like the drain in a sink—and some heart muscle dies.

There is no science to support this simple theory. The result of this bad science was dietary recommendations that actually increased the incidence of coronary artery disease from approximately 1960 to 2014 by recommending a high-carbohydrate diet. During these years, both the American Heart Association (AHA) and the U.S. Department of Agriculture (USDA) recommended a diet minimizing meat products and maximizing carbohydrates—fruits, vegetables, and whole grains. On January 1, 2012, Mark Bittman, a *New York Times* columnist, wrote, "…to eat better … the answer is known to everyone … eat more plants." On November 4, 1993, there was a television episode of *Seinfeld* with Mayor Rudy Giuliani regarding the horrors of finding fat in the non-fat yogurt. National Public Radio, on July 25, 2015, featured the Surgeon General of the U.S., Vivek Murthy, who reminded people to eat fruits and vegetables—no mention was made of protein or fat—just carbohydrates.

The demonization of dietary animal fats/saturated fats finds its origins in the work of Ancel Benjamin Keys. He and others found that cholesterol was the main ingredient in the blocked areas of the coronary arteries [20].

The idea that a low-fat, low-cholesterol diet would prove to prevent heart disease seems reasonably logical but has never been scientifically proven in ethnographic population studies nor in prospective studies.

Current evidence does not support cardiovascular guidelines that encourage high consumption of polyunsaturated fatty acids and low consumption of total saturated fats [21]. It is very difficult today to do large population prospective studies for a variety of reasons: it's difficult to control human dietary choices; it's difficult to prevent changes in diet over time; and it's difficult to define low-fat and high-fat diets in different countries. The famous Mediterranean diet had all of these problems yet concluded that there is something favorably affecting the lower incidence of coronary artery disease in the Mediterranean populations of Greece and Italy [22].

Approximately 50 years ago, Keys and colleagues described strikingly low rates of coronary heart disease in the Mediterranean region, where fat intake was relatively high but largely from olive oil. Controlled feeding of high-cholesterol and high-fat diets has shown that, compared to carbohydrates, both monounsaturated and polyunsaturated fats reduce LDL and triglycerides and increase HDL cholesterol—thus being beneficial and contrary to what Keys predicted [23]. Keys selected to study only six countries and excluded many countries for arbitrary reasons.

The Nurses' Health Study of 78,788 women clearly demonstrated that trans fat from partially hydrogenated vegetable oils (absent in traditional Mediterranean diets) was most strongly related to the risk of coronary artery disease. Polyunsaturated and monounsaturated fat were inversely associated with risk and were thus healthy [24].

Why dietary fat is rarely mentioned in the media as beneficial, despite objective scientific studies, remains a mystery. Who controls our cultural knowledge?

Accurate dietary population studies have been conducted in a 10,000-square-mile area of Kenya and Tanzania, where the Maasai tribe lives. The Maasai have few dietary choices, and their regular diet is 66% fat and consists almost entirely of cow's blood, milk and meat. Their serum cholesterol and beta-lipoprotein levels are low. The proof of the principle is that post-mortem dissection of their coronary arteries shows almost no coronary artery disease, and electrocardiograms (EKG or ECG) of the men show no evidence of old heart attacks (myocardial infarctions) [26].

An important additional finding was that Maasai men weigh less and have lower blood pressure levels than American and European men. The Maasai have body weights and blood pressure levels that remain nearly constant as they age, unlike American men, who nearly always gain weight and have higher blood pressure as they age.

Healthy fats consist of whole eggs, tree nuts, olive oil, seeds, nut oils, avocados, and ground tree-nut butter. Avoid commercial nut butters that have added sugar. All hydrogenated oils contain trans fats and must be avoided (canola oil).

The saturated fat present in meat and dairy products is essential and healthy. However, the total calorie content of your diet is still a limiting factor in food choices. Please avoid drinking milk, since it is unusually insulinogenic, and the calories do count.

Carbohydrates in Your Diet

Healthy carbohydrates include all vegetables and all berries. Other fruits including bananas, grapes, figs, and dates contain too much sugar. It's important to have vegetables or salads as often as you like—every day—to ensure sufficient fiber.

Unhealthy carbohydrates have a high glycemic index, meaning they contain sugars and raise blood glucose levels quickly, and so raise insulin levels quickly and therefore produce body fat quickly. Examples include any food with added sugar, soft drinks, any juice, pasta, pancakes, waffles, bread, pastry, cake, pie, cookies, ice cream, sorbet, candy, and most cold cereals. We've already discussed the glycemic index earlier in this book.

Carbohydrates and insulin are also essential for your body. Insulin is necessary for storing glycogen in your liver and in muscle cells, in addition to storing fat in fat cells. All of your cells need energy from sugar. This is where calories count, and we get fat and unhealthy only when we consume more calories than we burn.

In the presence of adequate protein, low-carbohydrate diets and high-carbohydrate diets give similar weight loss results [28]. Muscle growth improves in the presence of insulin [29].

Very low-carbohydrate diets raise serum cortisol levels and lower testosterone levels, resulting in fatigue and less muscle growth [30].

The question of, What is the best amount of carbohydrates for you, has been discussed earlier, and the amount will vary based on your goals, body shape (% body fat), and exercise intensity. **You need some carbohydrates.**

Foods Best Avoided

You shouldn't eat any man-made products, nor any food, when you don't know its ingredients.

Alcohol

Alcohol has been reported to have positive health benefits in the past. Moderate alcohol intake decreased the risk of coronary artery disease by 40% to 70% based on multiple epidemiological studies [31]. These studies were not randomized nor prospective and had different definitions of a standard drink and what is moderate. These studies were done using questions answered by patients filling out surveys. These 34 studies were grouped together in what is called a meta-analysis. The conclusion of these 34 studies involving over one million subjects was that alcohol drinkers have less risk of dying from a heart attack. A standard drink in the United States is 14 to 15 grams of alcohol. This is 12 ounces of beer, 5 ounces of wine, or 1.5 ounces of 80 proof liquor. More than two standard drinks per day in women and three drinks per day in men however did increase risk of dying. Similar results have been found in peripheral vascular disease and stroke. Stroke is an event in which the blood supply to a part of the brain is occluded, and brain cells die. The French paradox refers to the low incidence of coronary artery mortality in a country with a high incidence of smoking and a high consumption of saturated fat. The theory to explain the French lower-than-expected coronary heart disease was the high consumption of red wine [32]. Other studies do not confirm a specific alcoholic beverage type as better in coronary artery health, but all studies show that the amount of alcohol is important. In summary, moderate alcohol consumption defined as two standard drinks per day for men, lowers HDL-C, triglycerides, C-reactive protein, platelet aggregation, and fibrinogen level [33]. These blood test measurements were not long term, and longevity was not a measured outcome.

Achieving a balance between the health risks and benefits of alcohol consumption remains difficult, as each person has a different susceptibility to the adverse health consequences associated with alcohol consumption—addiction, dementia, cirrhosis, hypertension, diabetes, cardiomyopathy, congestive heart failure, and bone marrow suppression. Among participants 30–59 years of age and free of hypertension, diabetes, or cardiovascular disease, the lowest death rate was found with a consumption of less than one drink daily. **More recent and objective studies contradict any beneficial effects of alcohol.** Moderate consumption of alcohol over 30 years is associated with hippocampal (brain) atrophy, identical to Alzheimer's Disease [34]. Light drinking is associated with minimally increased risk of overall cancer [35]. For non-smoking men who are light drinkers, the cancer risk is not increased. For non-smoking women, the risk of cancer—especially breast cancer—increases with one alcoholic drink per day [35]. Owing to the objective evidence for brain damage, I do not drink alcohol, and I recommend no more than two alcoholic beverages per week.

Misunderstood Foods

The least understood and most controversial food is saturated fat—the fat found in dairy and red meat. Over the years, data has revealed that dietary saturated fatty acids (saturated fats) are not associated with coronary artery disease. Smoothies are smooth because the fiber has been broken down. Juicing or smoothies are thus not as healthy as the original ingredients when eaten individually. Fruit juice is just sugar (fructose and glucose), water, and some vitamins. It's best to take a multivitamin and avoid the sugar.

There are six artificial sweeteners in foods today: sucralose, saccharin, aspartame, acesulfame potassium, neotame, and Luo han guo extract. If you believe in Pavlov, diet soda should be bad for you—but I will admit that I still drink an occasional Diet Coke. With the artificial sweeteners, your tongue and mouth taste receptors stimulate the release of insulin and glucagon-like peptide [GLP-1]. The brain senses sugar, and the pancreas releases more insulin [36] [37, 16]. Artificial sweeteners also alter the bacteria in your GI tract—the microbiome. You already know that higher insulin levels create more body fat and can lead to leptin resistance.

Despite what critics say, caffeine can be healthy. Early studies showing coffee as harmful were done when the harmful effects of smoking were not taken into consideration, and most coffee drinkers in the past also smoked cigarettes.

According to the Mayo Clinic, coffee may protect you from Parkinson's disease, diabetes, and liver cancer. Coffee improves cognitive function, memory, and decreases the risk of depression by blocking the inhibitory neurotransmitter adenosine [38].

Caffeine is a fat burner and can increase adrenaline levels and release fatty acids from the fat tissues. Coffee can increase your metabolic rate by 3–11% [39].

A cup of coffee can improve your performance in the gym by 11–12% [40].

Milk has an unusually high insulin response that is greater than predicted by its carbohydrate content. Milk proteins—lactose, leucine, other amino acids—increase insulin by increasing the production of GLP-1 (glucagon-like peptide-1) by the cells of the small intestine [41]. Most milk products should be avoided in order to decrease your insulin levels and decrease your body fat. The exception to this is the time period when you are exercising to build muscle and the immediate hour after you complete your resistance training. This is the time your insulin will drive nutrients into your muscle cells for growth and repair. **After exercise is the time you need your post-workout branch chain amino acids and protein shake—milk proteins, whey protein, and simple carbohydrates. This is the only time you should eat simple carbs and milk products.**

Not all fruits are healthy. Fruit contains fructose, which can only be metabolized by the liver. This can lead to metabolic syndrome. If enough fiber is present—such as in berries—the damage is less. Bananas, dates, grapes, and figs have excessive sugar and contain insufficient fiber and thus should be avoided.

Wheat products should be avoided—bread, most cereals, and pasta. Wheat products are high-glycemic carbohydrates and by themselves raise insulin levels. **All wheat products contain gluten.** Gluten is a vegetable protein that interferes with the cells of the gastrointestinal tract and **stimulates an inflammatory response to a varying degree in all humans.** Gluten cannot be digested and blocks the activity of leptin. Leptin, as you may recall, is released by fat cells and tells your body to burn fat and stop eating. Known leptin blockers include insulin, artificial sweeteners, gluten, and the seasoning monosodium glutamate (MSG).

Eat all the vegetables and salads that you like. The energy required to digest salads and vegetables equals the added calories. The fiber is the real value of salads and vegetables. The magic of fiber is its ability to slow absorption of all other foods in the mix and decrease insulin levels.

There is no substitute for single-source real food that occurs in nature. When in doubt, read the label. Any box or can of food with a label contains processed products that do not occur normally in nature and contain added sugar. **"Heart healthy" may not be healthy for you, such as is the case of most boxed cereals. The definition of "heart healthy" is low sodium and low fat.** True heart healthy should measure sugar.

Metabolic syndrome is a modern disease associated with man-made food. You've been raised on and have become accustomed to eating processed, man-made food. It's time to stop eating this stuff and restore your body to good health. Don't listen to the advertisements that market foods. Few, if any, of these unnatural, man-made products are healthy.

Misunderstood Dieting

According to Dr. T. Mann [42], one-third to two-thirds of obese dieters regain more weight than they lost on their diets. **A low-calorie diet alone, without any other intervention or change, will usually fail and not lead to a health benefit.** The reason

94

for this is the change in circulating hormones that control body metabolism and hunger [43]. With caloric restriction alone in obese patients, many gastrointestinal hormones change, including a decrease in leptin and an increase in ghrelin, resulting in an increase in appetite, and these changes persist for over one year. The brain detects the decline in energy stores and decreases the metabolic rate to maintain homeostasis [44]. What is needed for a long-term health benefit is a change in the brain's set point for homeostasis. We must emphasize that **there is no evidence that dieting alone results in significant health improvements in the long term, regardless of initial weight change [45]. Do not despair; there is a solution, so continue reading.**

Processed Foods

Processed foods are not as healthy as foods obtained directly from plants or animals. Processed foods have additives such as preservatives, sugar, oil, salt, and are packaged, canned, or bottled. Minimally processed foods have nothing added to the food. Processed foods have been categorized into four groups by a complex classification system called NOVA. The definitions vary, but in general group 1 is unprocessed or minimally processed food; group 2 foods have small amounts of food industry ingredients added for seasoning or flavor; group 3 foods are industrially manufactured foods with two or three additives made from foods; group 4 foods are ultra-processed foods that may contain non-food additives. Fast food is ultra-processed. The important point is that the food additives in ultra-processed foods may cause metabolic problems. Fast foods have ingredients that increase the appetite and cause over-eating when compared with unprocessed foods [46]. The preservative propionate found in many ultra-processed foods causes insulin resistance in humans. This may be the reason many fast food consumers are obese.

CHAPTER 10
Summary of Essential Information About Food—What Exactly You Should Eat

The Most Important Choices of Your Life

You choose food for many different reasons. Some of these reasons are based upon your knowledge of **"what is healthy to eat."** Most Americans are not healthy in that they are overweight and have or will soon have chronic metabolic diseases, including hypertension, type 2 diabetes, and small blood vessel disease, including dementia, impotence, coronary artery disease, and renal dysfunction. These chronic metabolic diseases are preventable with exercise and a healthy diet. The purpose of this essay is to provide science-based information about food. Everyone thinks they know what is healthy to eat, yet few people are optimally healthy. Much of our popular culture food information is incorrect [1]. This essay will focus on the latest positive scientific studies and attempt to define what exactly is healthy to eat. Much of this information has already been discussed, but it is so important that it is worth summarizing in one place.

Meat

Red meat contains saturated fat, omega-6 fats, and omega-3 fats. Despite popular culture, studies of over 600,000 people have found no link between saturated fat and heart disease [2]. Meat is the best source of protein and amino acids for muscle maintenance and muscle growth. The protein found in meat is better than the protein found in vegetables [3]. Vegetable proteins lack leucine. The protein content of 4 ounces of beef is equivalent to 3 cups of lentils. In simple terms, **eating meat will not cause cardio-vascular disease, i.e., it will not clog your arteries.** Part of the incorrect thinking about meat and saturated fat were studies that focused on total cholesterol levels and total LDL blood tests. Total cholesterol levels are not a measure of heart health. Saturated fat does raise total LDL bad cholesterol. LDL, however, is composed of large particles and small particles. Only the small particle LDL is bad, and saturated fat raises mostly large particle LDL [4]. LDL subsets were not measured in the past studies, giving rise to the theory that saturated fat was bad. The dangerous small particle LDL is increased by dietary sugar and in high-carbohydrate diets [5]. Unfortunately, high-carbohydrate low-fat diets have been recommended recently by physicians and the U.S. governmental agencies without any scientific evidence [6]. Because this is most important, please remember that **the largest and most recent scientific medical study to prevent heart disease found that saturated fat diets do not cause heart disease [7]. In addition, excess dietary protein not utilized to build or repair tissues will be converted to glucose—glucose neogenesis—and this is not healthy.**

Processed Meat

Processed meat includes any meat that has been modified to prolong shelf life or change taste. Examples include bacon, ham, sausage, salami, baloney, hot dogs, and many other cold cuts and canned meats. The processes include smoking, salting, curing, and marinating. The preservative sodium nitrate is frequently added to prevent bacterial growth. In 2015, the World Health Organization found that eating 50 grams of processed meat daily (one hot dog or 4 strips of bacon) increased the incidence of colon cancer by 18 percent [8]. This means that **the real risk of getting colon cancer in your lifetime would go from 5% to 6%, and you would need to eat a hot dog equivalent every day. However, processed foods contain non-food additives that have been shown to increase appetite and increase insulin resistance. AVOID PROCESSED FOODS—ESPECIALLY FAST FOOD.**

Vegetable Plant-Based Food

Studies comparing vegetarians to meat eaters often contain an inherent flaw. People who are very focused on their diet and avoid eating much red meat frequently will exercise more, do not smoke nor drink, and have a very healthy lifestyle. A large population-based study of 245,000 people found no difference in all-cause mortality in vegetarians and meat eaters [9].

Vegetables do not contain all the vitamins and minerals that you need. Plants are not good sources for vitamin A, omega-3 fatty acids, vitamin D, vitamin B12, iron, and calcium. Vegetables are carbohydrates for energy and the best source of fiber for your digestive tract. There are essential fats and essential proteins that you must eat to be healthy and that cannot be synthesized by your body, but there are no essential carbohydrates. **There are many**

health benefits from eating fiber. Fiber slows the absorption of nutrients in your small intestine and lowers your peak insulin levels, resulting in less synthesis of body fat and lowers the risk for type 2 diabetes, coronary artery disease, and colon cancer [10].

Fruit

The high sugar content of most fruits is problematic for most Americans because 60 percent or more of Americans are overweight or obese, and the incidence of type 2 diabetes is increasing [11]. Dried fruits like figs, dates, and raisins have the highest sugar content and should be avoided. The fresh fruits with high sugar content in descending order include raisins, figs, bananas, grapes, cherries, mangoes, kiwis, pineapples, apples, blueberries, nectarines, watermelons, oranges, and apricots. **Berries have the least sugar and the most fiber of all the fruits and are the healthiest fruits to eat.**

Amazing Fat Facts

We have already discussed that fats are a necessary and essential part of your diet. **Fats do one thing that no other macronutrient can do—they increase our metabolic rate.** A diet of 60 percent fat, 30 percent protein and 10 percent carbohydrate will burn 300 more calories per day than a diet of 60 percent carbohydrate, 20 percent protein, and 20 percent fat in the same participants [12]. Fats will make you healthier by helping you lose body fat, maintain more muscle while dieting, lower your inflammatory molecules, increase your HDL, lower your triglyceride blood levels, and decrease your markers of inflammation [13]. The simple truth is that high-fat low-carbohydrate diets are best for healthy weight loss [14]. The biggest nutritional mistake made by medical societies and the U.S. government agencies was to recommend a low-fat high-carbohydrate diet for over 40 years and cause a nationwide increase in obesity that continues today [15]. Not all fats are healthy. The monounsaturated fats from plants and animals such as nut oils, olive oils, avocados, nuts, butter, lard, and chicken fat can be healthy. **The monounsaturated fat in canola oil is very unhealthy.** When fat is exposed to high temperatures, it can become unhealthy [16].

There are two essential polyunsaturated fats—omega-3 and omega-6 fatty acids. Both are essential in a ratio 1 to 1. Omega-3 fatty acids are found in seafood, eggs, meat, flax seed, and walnuts. Omega-6 fatty acids are found in nuts, seeds, grains, beans, and some vegetable oils. Omega-6 fatty acids are used in many processed foods and snacks made with canola oil, soybean oil, corn oil, and their overuse will decrease your life expectancy [17]. Omega-6 fatty acids eaten in excess were studied in a prospective randomized study of 9000 hospitalized and, thus, well-controlled patients. The experimental group was fed polyunsaturated fats from corn oil exclusively (increased Omega-6), while the control group was fed saturated animal fats as well as some polyunsaturated fats. **The experimental group on polyunsaturated fats had a significant decrease in serum total cholesterol levels yet a 22% increase in mortality.** Systematic review for corroborating information identified five randomized controlled trials showing that cholesterol lowering, unsaturated fat interventions had no evidence of benefit on mortality from coronary heart disease [18]. The following fats are not healthy: Crisco, fake butter, margarine, hydrogenated soybean or vegetable oil, trans fat.

Medium chain triglycerides (MCT) is an amazing fat supplement. It is present in coconut oil and available as a food supplement. MCT, when ingested, goes directly to your liver and can be used by cells as an energy source without storage in fat cells. MCT increases your metabolic rate and increases body fat loss [19].

Legumes—Beans

Beans are the dry seeds of some plants and are not vegetables. Beans contain vitamins, minerals, and sufficient nutrients to generate a new plant. Beans are mostly carbohydrates. They also contain lectins, which protect plants from being eaten, because they cause human intestinal cell dysfunction and physical discomfort [20]. Bean protein is low in leucine and less efficient in building muscle compared to animal protein or whey protein.

Grains

Grains are grass seeds. The outer layer of the grain is bran and is undigestible fiber that decreases the absorption of nutrients and lowers insulin levels. Fiber is healthy. The germ of the grain contains vitamins, minerals, protein, and a little fat. The remaining endosperm is carbohydrates—high glycemic starch which increases insulin levels and is stored in your body as fat. Remember that carbohydrates are not essential for your health. Grains historically were cultivated by people to make a stable source of man-made food.

Grains contain lectins, and the lectin gluten interferes with the cells in the small bowel and activates the gut immune system against the intestinal cells. This is an auto-immune inflammatory response causing varying degrees of dysfunctions—leaky gut syndrome to celiac disease [21]. Gluten can be tolerated by most healthy people, but it is best avoided when possible.

Breakfast cereals, including oatmeal, are popular foods that are mostly sugar and should be avoided. **Many children start their day with cereal, and many children are becoming obese in the USA [22].** In a major study, overweight children were fed one of three possible breakfasts with the same calorie content: eggs, instant oatmeal, or steel-cut oatmeal. With the egg breakfast, children had lower blood sugars, lower insulin levels, lower cortisol levels, and ate less food the rest of the day [23]. Protein and fat are healthier foods than grain. Some grains do not greatly elevate blood sugar, such as quinoa and amaranth, and are healthy to eat.

Diet Soda—Artificial Sweeteners

Diet soda and artificial sweeteners increase insulin production and, thus, increase body fat [24].

Summary

1. **Meat is healthy as long as you use the protein to build muscle or repair tissues.**

2. **Saturated fat does not cause heart disease.**

3. **Vegetables are healthy—fiber is important.**

4. **The best fruits are berries.**

5. **A high-fat low-carbohydrate diet is best for weight loss.**

6. **Olive oil, coconut oil, and mct are healthy.**

7. **Beans and grains are not essential foods.**

8. **Glutin can cause digestive problems in many people.**

9. **Artificial sweeteners increase body fat.**

10. **Fast food or any ultra-processed food accelerates body fat production, weight gain, and obesity.**

CHAPTER 11
Fiber in Your Diet is Amazing

Fiber in your diet is essential for optimal body function. This is new and exciting information that redefines the role of fiber. In the past, fiber has been described as indigestible plant carbohydrates that kept your bowel movements regular. We do not digest fiber, but your gut bacteria needs fiber. Think of your gut bacteria as an essential organ the size of one kidney and more metabolically active than your liver. Our gut bacteria ferments fiber and produces short chain fatty acids that are absorbed through the large intestine (colon) into the blood stream and affects our hormones, metabolism, body fat, and our immune system. The study of our ancient ancestors and current hunter-gatherer's diet [8] reveals that our ancestors ate much more fiber than we do today.

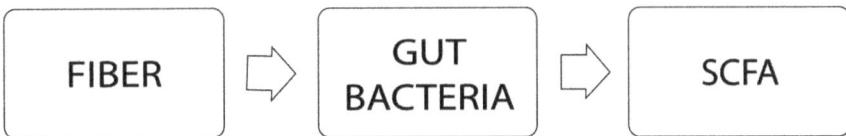

FIBER ⇨ GUT BACTERIA ⇨ SCFA

Fiber and Weight Loss

Fiber mechanically slows the absorption of calories, lowers peak insulin levels and stimulates the stretch receptors of the gastrointestinal tract. Fiber can trap fat and prevent fat absorption by increasing the fat in our stool. The overall result is a 10% decrease in effective calories and weight loss [1][2]. In addition, the increased smooth muscle activity in the small intestine caused by increased fiber decreases blood glucose levels [3]. Leptin, as you may remember, is a hormone produced by fat cells that tells our brain to stop eating. Fiber increases SCFA, and SCFA increases leptin [4]. Leptin blood levels qualitatively measure total body fat and do not change quickly from meal to meal. There are two other hormones that act rapidly from meal to meal to decrease appetite-PYY and GLP-1. SCFA increases production of both PYY and GLP-1 [5]. The hunger hormone ghrelin is suppressed by fiber as well [6].

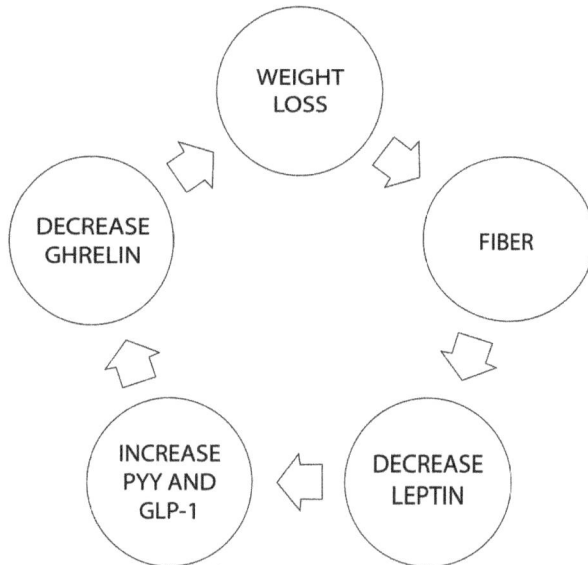

WEIGHT LOSS

FIBER

DECREASE LEPTIN

INCREASE PYY AND GLP-1

DECREASE GHRELIN

Dietary Fiber Causes Weight Loss Through the Hormones That Control Hunger

Food With Fiber

In the United States, people who eat more fiber are less likely to become obese [7]. The recommended daily amount of fiber for adults is 25 grams for women and 38 grams for men. It is likely that even more fiber than this is helpful. Foods that contain fiber are fruits and vegetables. There is no fiber in meat nor dairy. Below is a list of high-fiber foods—stars indicate lower calories. Berries are the best high-fiber, low-calorie fruits.

Pears—3.1 (grams of fiber per 100 grams of fruit)

Strawberries*—2 (grams of fiber per 100 grams of fruit)

Avocado—6.7

Apple—2.4

Raspberries*—6.5

Carrots—2.8 (grams of fiber per 100 grams of vegetable)

Beets—2.8

Broccoli*—2.6

Artichoke*—8.6

Brussels Sprouts*—2.6

Lentils—7.9

Kidney Beans—6.4

Split Peas—8.3

Chickpeas—7.6

Oats—10.6

Popcorn*—14.5

Almonds—12.5

Sweet Potatoes—2.5

Dark Chocolate—10.9.

CHAPTER 12
Exercise

The Benefits of Exercise, the Missing Ingredient: Metabolic Role of Exercise

We will define exercise, for our purposes, as physical activity requiring effort designed to improve health. Exercise can be designed to improve endurance, strength, balance and flexibility. Even a small amount of daily exercise will make you live longer [1]. In chapter 22, we will discuss senescent cells, exercise, and longevity.

Exercise is the missing ingredient in most unhealthy lifestyles. In my opinion, this chapter is the most important part of this book. **Exercise and diet restrictions can reverse the metabolic syndrome and reset the brain's set point.** Epidemiological studies reveal a higher incidence of metabolic syndrome in people who don't exercise [2]. Supervised long-term, intense exercise raises high-density lipoprotein (HDL), lowers triglycerides, and reduces blood pressure. Both diet and exercise are required to lower insulin resistance [3] and can completely reverse/cure type 2 diabetes.

The majority of insulin stimulated glucose uptake occurs in skeletal muscle where the glucose is stored as glycogen [10]. This means that if you have muscle or are building muscle, you are less likely to develop insulin resistance, type 2 diabetes, metabolic syndrome, and cardiovascular disease. Skeletal muscle is crucial for glucose metabolism. Both endurance and resistance exercise improve insulin sensitivity. Muscle cells, like fat cells, are secretory and produce myokines that improve metabolism. One example is irisin, which promotes the development of brown fat from white fat and increases thermogenesis instead of fat storage—increasing lean body mass.

There are two broad categories of exercise. Cardiovascular exercises (endurance training—ET) are aimed at improving the heart, lungs, and circulation. Resistance training (RT) exercises are designed to strengthen and build muscles. **Cardiovascular interval training is superior to continuous moderate cardiovascular exercise** for enhancing endothelial function, improving insulin signaling, lowering blood glucose levels, and deceasing lipogenesis in adipose tissue. Both resistance training and cardiovascular aerobic exercise are equally effective for weight loss and lowering blood pressure [4]. Resistance training builds new muscle.

The benefits of exercise are observable inside the skeletal muscle cells with an **increase in the size and number of mitochondria [5].**

Exercise builds muscle, and it's the *only* way one can build muscle. Aging and the associated decline in muscle capacity are associated with a decline in mitochondria content and function. A similar mitochondria decline is seen in insulin resistance and maturity onset diabetes [6]. Exercise increases the number of mitochondria in cells, and these new mitochondria then burn more energy with greater efficiency. The cells in the liver produce less visceral fat [7].

Exercise decreases both glucose and insulin levels, and with proper diet, can reverse insulin resistance. Exercise will improve the brain's response to leptin and decrease cortisol levels. The best treatment for stress relief and insomnia is exercise.

The American Heart Association recommends both ET and RT for both people with *and* without heart disease [8]. Both RT (weightlifting) and ET (running, swimming, jogging, biking) improve health, but each has different benefits.

With regard to body composition, both types of exercise increase bone mineral density and prevent bone loss and fracture. ET is better for increasing body fat loss, while RT increases muscle mass and strength, thus increasing lean body mass. Both are equally effective with regard to glucose metabolism, insulin levels, and sensitivity. Both are nearly equally effective for lipid control; ET has a slight advantage in lowering triglycerides. ET is clearly superior for cardiovascular dynamics—lower resting heart rate, cardiac output, and cellular oxygen consumption (VO2 max). RT is better for increasing the basal metabolic rate. Both are equally effective for quality of life measures. **YOU NEED BOTH!**

REVERSES METABOLIC SYNDROME;
INCREASES INSULIN SENSITIVITY;
IMPROVES LEPTIN SIGNALING

RAISES GOOD HDL, AND LOWERS
TRIGLYCERIDES

DECREASES BLOOD PRESSURE

BUILDS MUSCLE AND INCREASES
STRENGTH

DECREASES STRESS

PROLONGS LIFE—ELIMINATES
SENESCENT CELLS

REDUCES C-REACTIVE PROTEIN

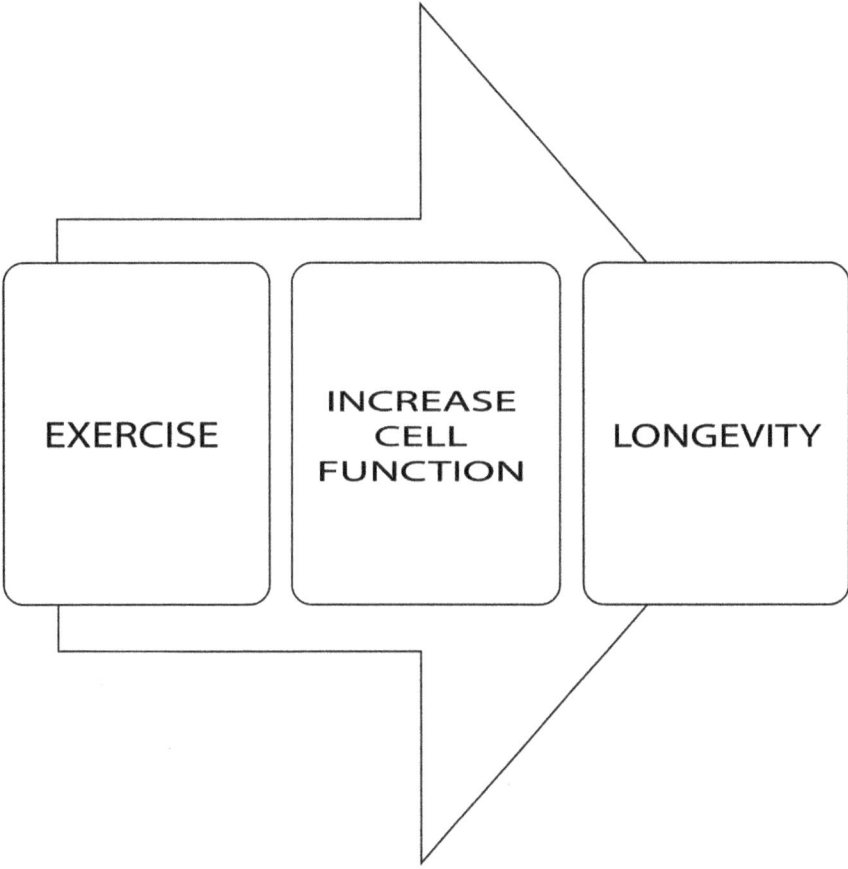

EXERCISE → INCREASE CELL FUNCTION → LONGEVITY

Both types of exercise are important. It's sad to see an obese person with a joint or bone injury that prevents their ability to exercise and limits their ability to prevent insulin resistance and the subsequent metabolic syndrome. In my opinion, diet and exercise over time will reset the brain's set point.

Obese people have a high fracture rate [9]. The benefits of exercise are short-lived, and thus exercises must be done frequently and regularly to maintain the beneficial effects. Exercise will restore your cells to a higher level of health, with efficient mitochondria and increased function.

As mentioned previously, exercise and diet can eliminate metabolic syndrome. You now have the basic scientific knowledge of how your body works. Would you like to know more? Do you want to know how to look and feel younger?

CHAPTER 13
How to be Strong, Robust, and Healthy

In this chapter, we'll discuss what science can tell us about muscle building. The assumption is that muscle strength at any age increases your activity level and improves your quality of life.

Exercise Will Lengthen Your Life and Improve Your Health

There is objective data indicating that **exercise will lengthen your life span [1].** The data is positive for all age groups, with results being most pronounced in men over 60 years of age. Vigorous exercise is even more beneficial [2]. This may appear to be obvious and logical, but it was not objectively proven until 1995.

The information in this book introducing you to exercise and disseminating knowledge regarding the body is based on scientific data. By implementing your newfound knowledge, you'll be able to change the way you look and feel.

Exercise will affect, in some way, every cell in your body. Your body will change when stressed by exercise, and it will adapt. This is referred to as Specific Adaption to the Imposed Demand (SAID) [3]. This is what exercise does. What form of exercise you choose will depend upon *you*—your abilities, your motivation, and your goals—*just you.*

Your body needs energy constantly, whether at rest or while exercising. We discussed this in the section on adenosine triphosphate (ATP) and mitochondria. The mitochondria are independent parts of the interior of cells, and they use oxygen and glucose to produce energy in the form of ATP.

Mitochondria are the engines inside cells. As mentioned earlier, **when you increase your exercise, your muscle cells adapt by increasing the number of mitochondria and producing more ATP [4]. When this occurs, you burn fat, and your muscles produce more force. You are now on your path to a healthy lifestyle.**

In time, and with patience and the knowledge gained from this book, you'll begin reshaping your body by burning fat and increasing muscle mass. The force of your muscle contractions will strengthen your bones. The heart muscles will enlarge and become more efficient in order to pump more blood to your skeletal muscles. The number of small blood vessels throughout your body will increase, and your brain will become more efficient. Your perceived stress, as measured by cortisol output, will decrease; you will sleep better and experience less anxiety and more energy; you will live longer. Exercise benefits every organ in your body.

Mental Health and Exercise

According to the National Institute of Mental Health, in 2013, there were approximately 10 million adults aged 18 or older in the U.S. who had some form of serious mental illness (SMI). This represented 4.2% of all U.S. adults [nimh.nih.gov]. A serious mental illness is defined as a mental, emotional or behavioral problem that results in impairment of lifestyle and meets the criteria specified in the *Diagnostic and Statistical Manual of Mental Disorders.*

In 2006, the Agency for Healthcare Research and Quality estimated the cost of SMI in the U.S. to be $57.5 billion, due solely to the loss of income.

Depression is a common illness, affecting at least 1 in 5 people during their lifetime. Exercise has been advocated as an adjunct to the usual treatment. A review and meta-analysis done by Cochrane identified all available randomized trials, which compared exercise with either no treatment or an established treatment. In 23 trials (907 participants), which compared exercise with no treatment or a control intervention, the data indicated a large clinical benefit. **Exercise did improve the symptoms of depression** [5].

The effects of aerobic and anaerobic exercise on anxiety levels, absenteeism, job satisfaction, and resting heart rate were investigated. Results indicated that aerobic subjects significantly reduced their anxiety levels over a single exercise session. Post-exercise anxiety decreased over eight weeks for both groups. There were no changes evident in job satisfaction, absenteeism, or resting heart rate.

These results show that **aerobic exercise is superior to anaerobic exercise for anxiety reduction** [6].

Insomnia

Pharmacotherapy in the form of sleeping pills is the most often prescribed treatment for insomnia. However, sleep aids carry side effects and may not be recommended for long-term treatment. Exercise may instead prove to be the treatment of choice [7, 8].

In one study, patients aged 50 to 76 years with moderate sleep complaints were randomized to either 16 weeks of moderate-intensity exercise training or a wait-listed control condition. Exercise consisted of four daily 30 to 40-minute periods of endurance training (low-impact aerobics or brisk walking) prescribed at 60% to 75% of maximal heart rate. **Patients in the exercise group showed significant improvement in sleep parameters of self-rated sleep quality [7].**

How Much Exercise is Enough?

Cardiovascular exercises include running, jogging, swimming, cycling, elliptical, and using the newer cardiovascular equipment. The relative intensity of cardiovascular exercise is easily measured by two simultaneous methods: the subjective talk test, and the objective measure of heart rate. It's easy to use a heart rate monitor, and many exercise devices have them built-in.

According to the Mayo Clinic, vigorous exercise occurs when your heart rate is 70% to 85% of your Maximum Heart Rate (MHR). This formula determines your MHR: 220 minus your age.

With vigorous activity, you won't be able to speak complete sentences due to being out of breath. This is a very simple definition of *vigorous*, but it's a measurable starting point for most active adults. Moderate intensity exercise is defined as 64% to 76% of your MHR. With moderate exercise, you can talk, but you cannot sing. The mathematic formula method of MHR determination isn't accurate for athletes who have ventricular hypertrophy with a slow baseline heart rate.

A more complicated approach, as recommended by the National Academy of Sports Medicine, defines Target Heart Rate =

(Maximum Heart Rate minus Resting Heart Rate) x Desired Intensity % + Resting Heart Rate [9].

The Centers for Disease Control and Prevention recommends 150 to 300 minutes per week of moderate cardiovascular exercise or 75 to 150 minutes of vigorous cardiovascular exercise. They also recommend two days of muscle-strengthening activities per week that address all major muscle groups. The muscle strengthening recommendations are not well described by the CDC nor by the Special Communication in the Journal of the American Medical Association [10].

Muscle building activities in general should involve weight or resistance training for each muscle group at least once a week. Each muscle should be exercised to failure once a week.

This training is the only path to increase the muscle mass that you're otherwise losing. Modern physical therapy science teaches us that before we can build muscle safely and efficiently, we must be flexible and have core strength.

High-Intensity Interval Training (HIIT)

High-intensity interval training is a type of endurance training involving short periods of maximal effort followed by periods of maintenance or recovery effort. What can differ is the timing and type of endurance exercise.

A typical cycling HIIT pattern may be four to six maximal (all-out) 30-second cycling sprints with each sprint session separated by four to five-minute recovery periods of comfortable cycling. When HIIT is compared to longer steady endurance training, the HIIT patterns show increased mitochondrial density in muscle cells and greater muscle performance improvements [11, 12, 13, 14]. This HIIT can be adapted to every type of cardiovascular aerobic exercise (walking, running, treadmill, elliptical machine, or bicycle).

When to Exercise: Morning, Afternoon, Evening?

There are conflicting scientific studies on the best time to do aerobic exercise. The results depend upon exercise time, intensity, and measured endpoint. There is no consensus. In regard to resistance training, again there are conflicting studies. The best time to exercise depends upon your individual daily schedule. In other words, the best time is up to you according to your schedule.

Exercise and Appetite

Exercise burns calories and increases body metabolism. It is logical that exercise should increase appetite. If we look at successful athletes such as long-distance runners and long-distance bicyclists, they usually have lean, muscular bodies. Can exercise decrease appetite? It turns out that in the presence of adequate muscle and liver glycogen (carbohydrate) stores, exercise does not increase appetite [15]. In order to build or increase muscle glycogen stores, you must first build muscle. In order to build and maintain liver glycogen stores, this requires exercise as well.

Chapter 14
The First Thing to do in the Gym

Flexibility and Warm-Up; Myofascial Release; Dynamic Stretching

Warming up before and after exercising has been studied in detail. This area of study has many variables and is quite complex. Flexibility is defined as the ability of skeletal muscles and tendons to lengthen. Muscles and tendons are covered with soft tissue called fascia, which provide tension and support. In response to injury or resistance training, fascia changes in tension and becomes less elastic [1]. The fascia will limit flexibility and range of motion unless it's manually stretched. Thus, it's important to first release the fascia by way of myofascial release or massage before exercising the muscle.

Static flexibility measures the range of motion of a joint. An example of static stretching is bending to touch your toes. Static stretching before exercising will not prevent injury or soreness, *and* it will make the muscle transiently weaker [2].

However, static stretching a muscle for 30 seconds on a regular basis will increase the range of motion of the muscle, and this is an important benefit [3].

The best time to perform static stretching is *after* the muscle

has been exercised, *not* before. Static stretching is not a good "warmup."

Dynamic stretching is the ideal warmup. Dynamic stretching involves a repetitive joint movement that increases in range with each repetition and increases body temperature. It's important to increase the flow of blood to the tendons and muscles you're about to exercise. It's also important for your brain to activate as many of the muscles that are involved in this joint movement as possible. Examples of dynamic stretching include knee bends, jumping jacks and jogging. There are many testimonials from athletic coaches published in the *Journal of Strength and Conditioning* which support this type of warmup.

The big picture is that flexibility, or increased range of motion, will improve if you perform myofascial release followed by light dynamic stretching before exercising and static stretching after you exercise. Myofascial release may also be beneficial after exercising.

WARM-UP
ROUTINE
BEFORE
EXERCISE

MYOFASCIAL RELEASE

DYNAMIC STRETCH

EXERCISE

Examples of Myofascial Release Using Foam Roller; Dynamic Stretching

Releasing Piriformis and Gluteus

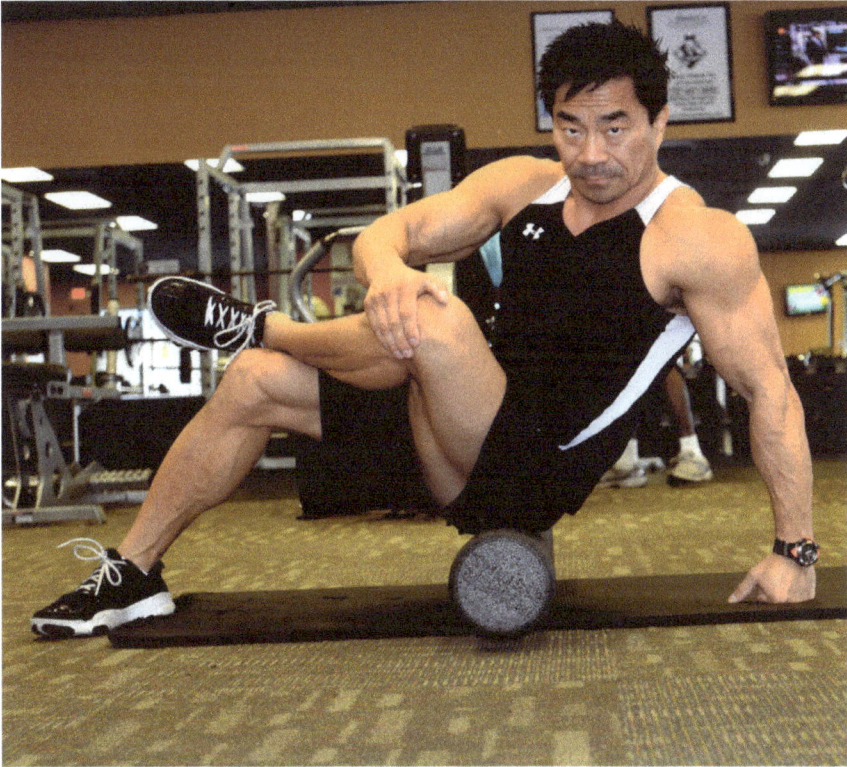

Relaxing Iliotibial Band

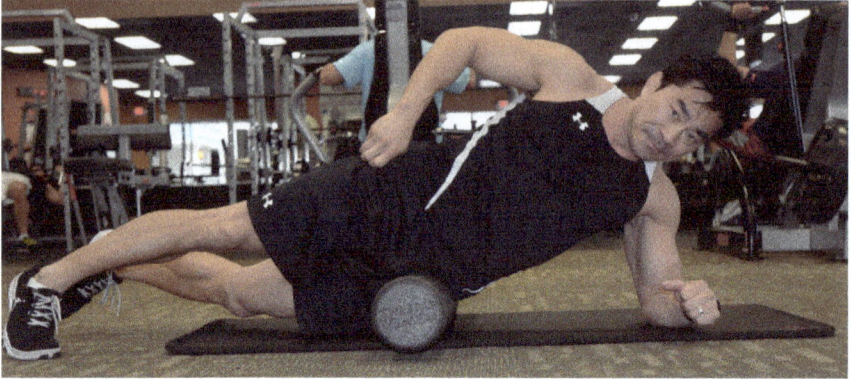

Releasing Adductors

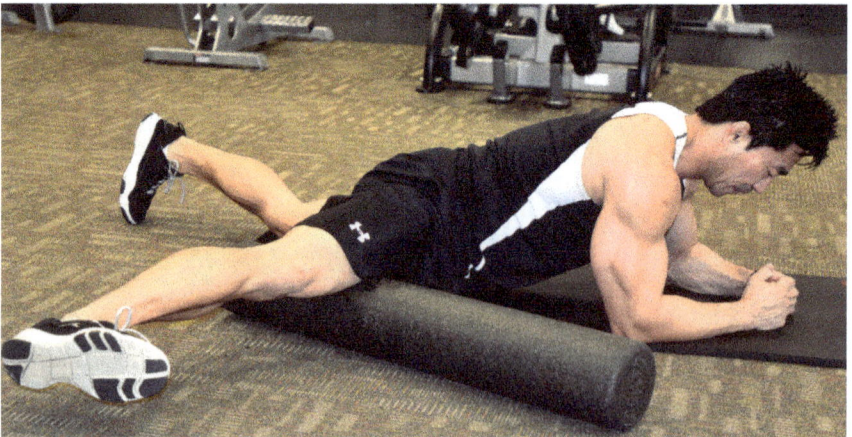

Releasing Calves

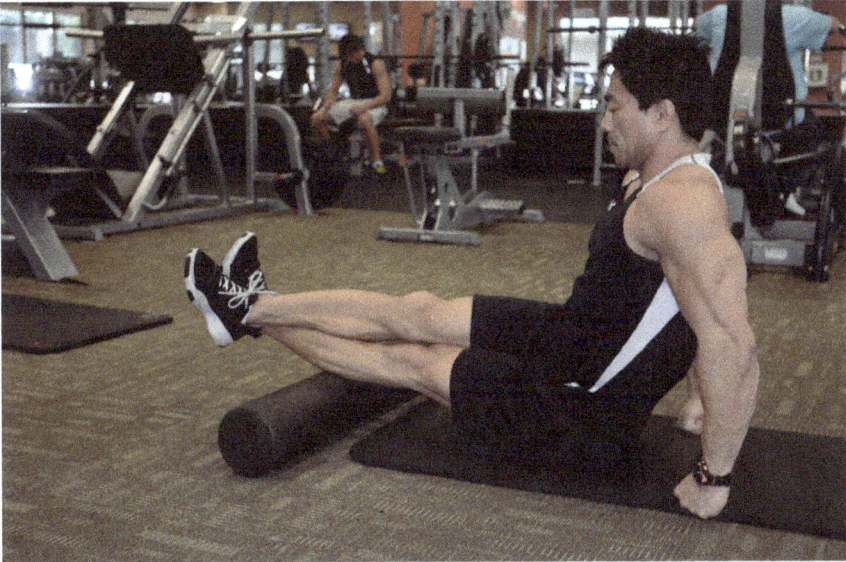

Myofascial release is an important part of each training day and can be done pre and post-exercise. It's an important part of any flexibility program as well as exercise recovery programs.

Releasing Latissimus Dorsi

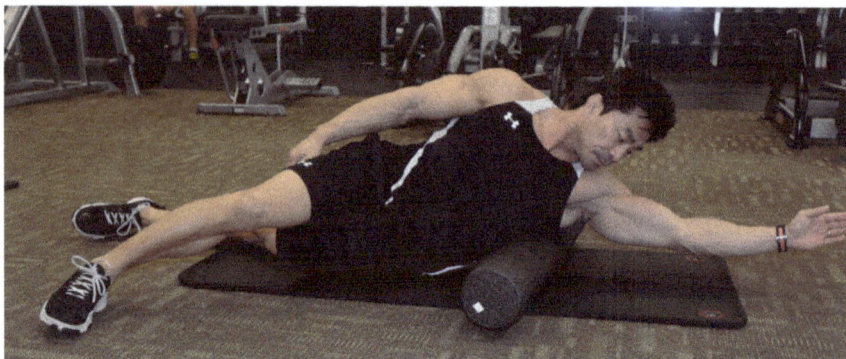

Releasing Erector Spinae

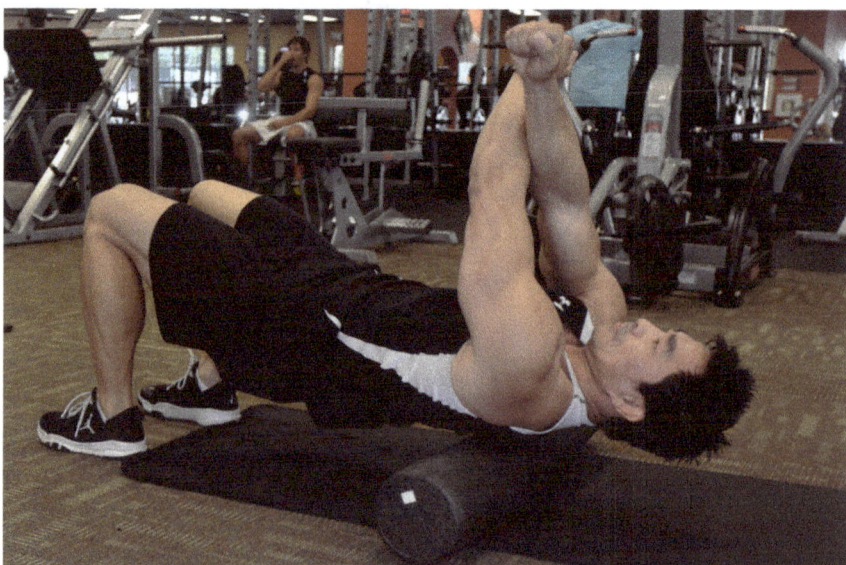

Dynamic Stretching:
Repetitive Joint Movement

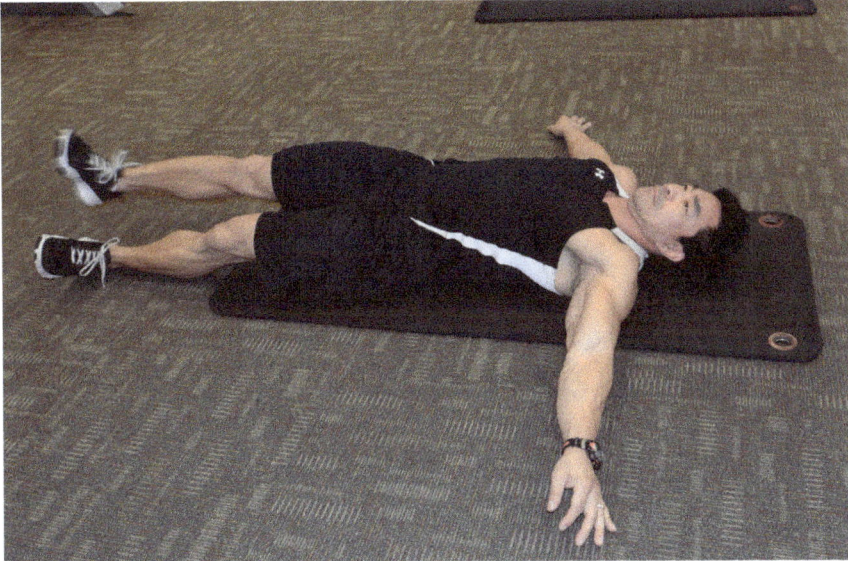

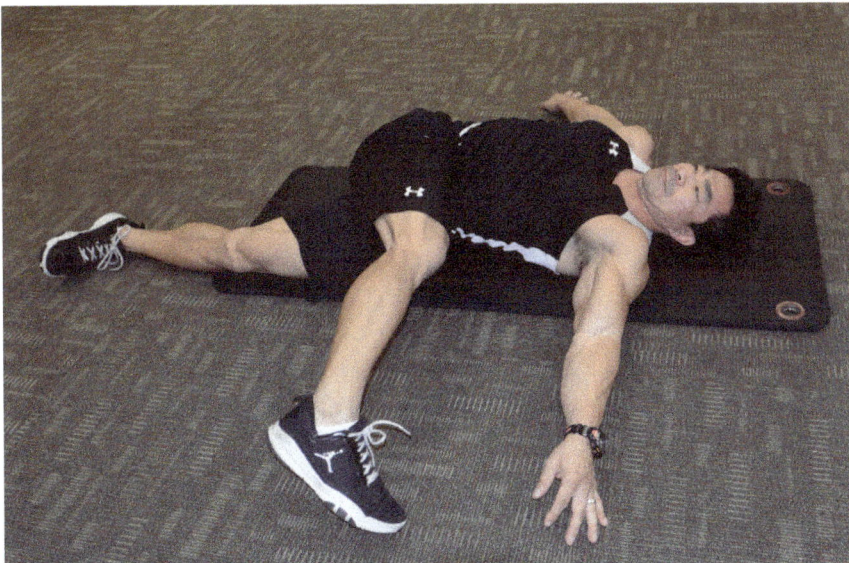

Dynamic Stretching

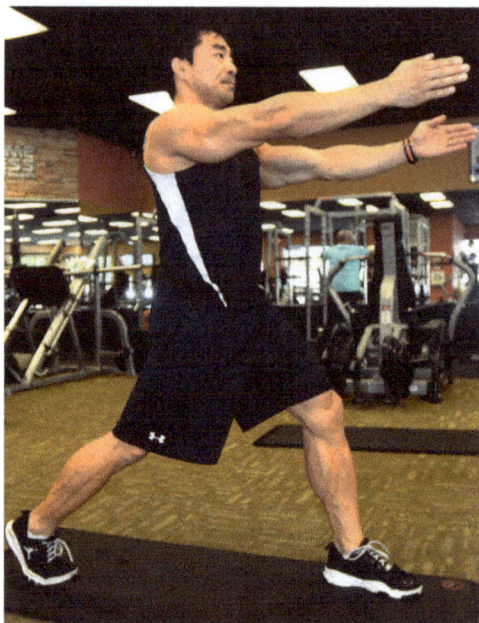

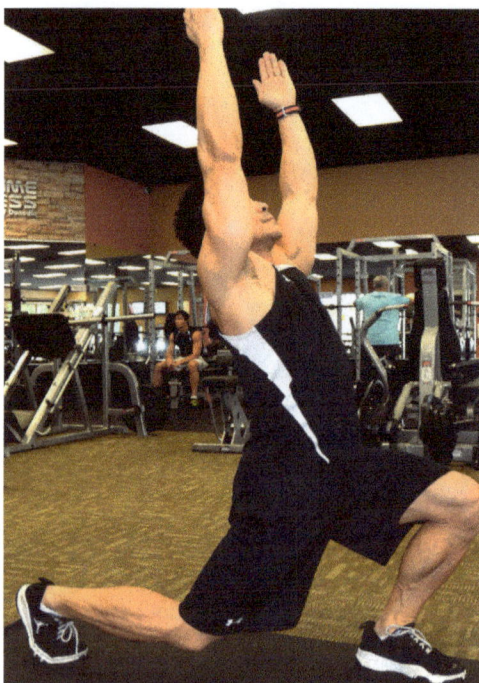

Dynamic Stretching

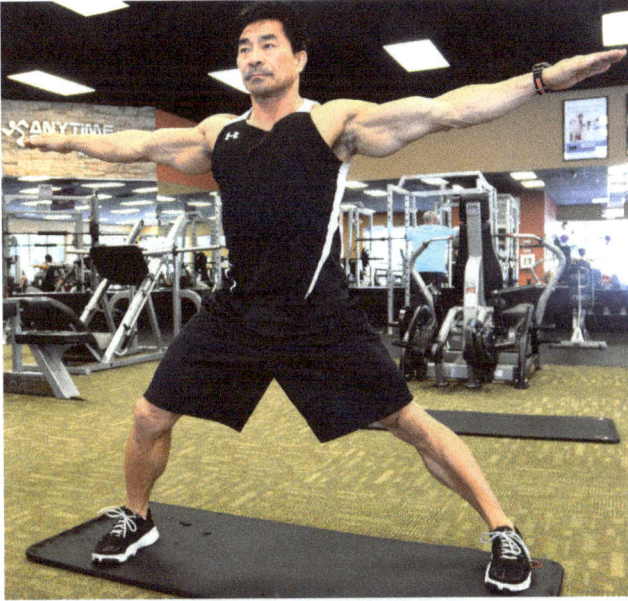

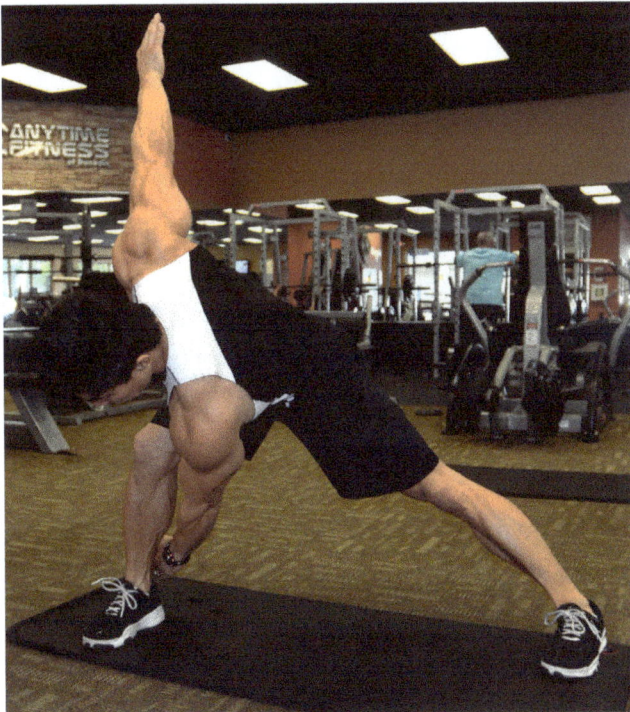

Dynamic Stretching

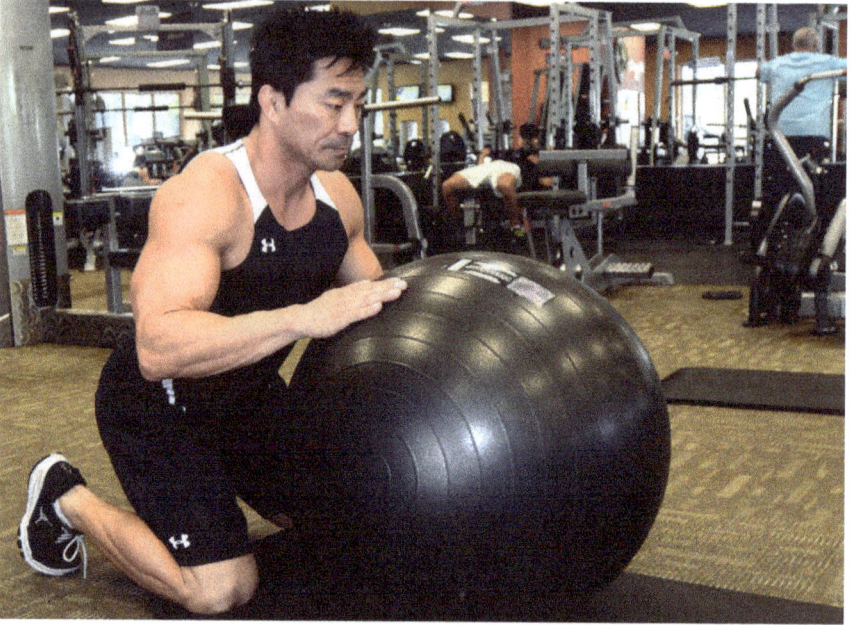

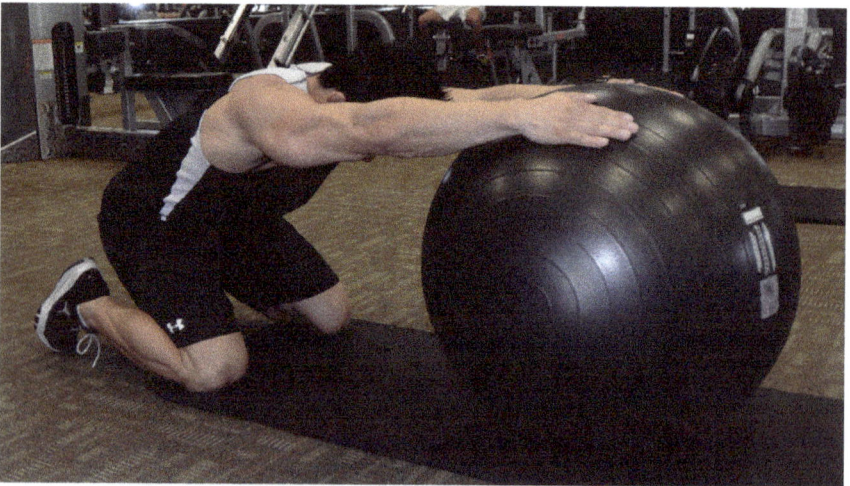

The Core—Your Most Important Muscles

The core muscles connect the arms and chest to the pelvis. Core muscles create stability between your upper and lower body when you perform complex movements such as running, lifting, and twisting. The core muscles align the spine, ribs, and pelvis and thus are the basis of one's posture. The major core muscles include the pelvic floor, the transverse abdominis, the internal and external obliques, the rectus abdominis, and all the muscles of the spine and buttocks.

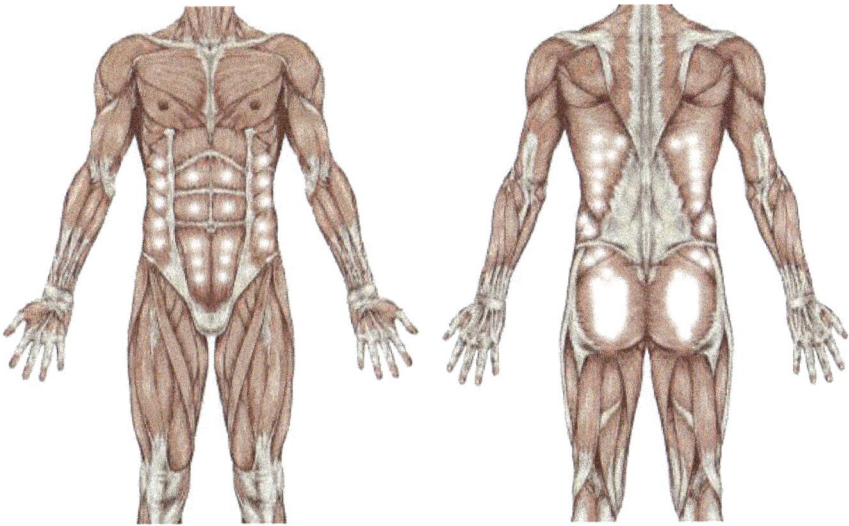

The above picture highlights some of the more visible anterior and posterior core muscles. Other internal core muscles, not visible above, are responsible for urinary and bowel continence.

Core muscles initiate all dynamic physical activities in nearly every sport. Many sports injuries, including those causing back pain, happen due to weak core muscles. Both yoga and Pilates improve core stability and can be a very important part of your exercise program.

Examples of Core Exercises

Core Exercise #1: The Plank

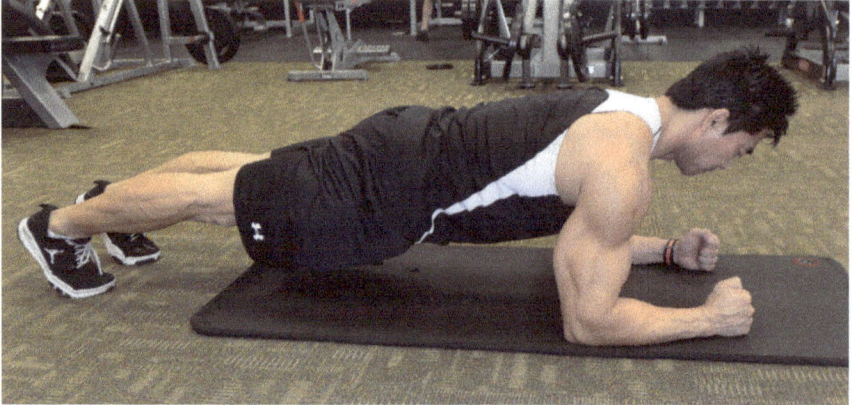

Core Exercise #2

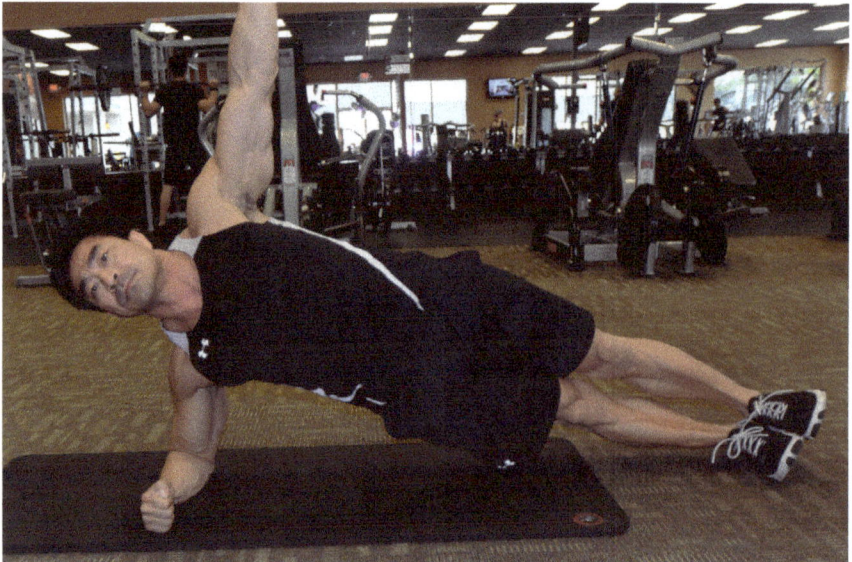

Core Exercise #3

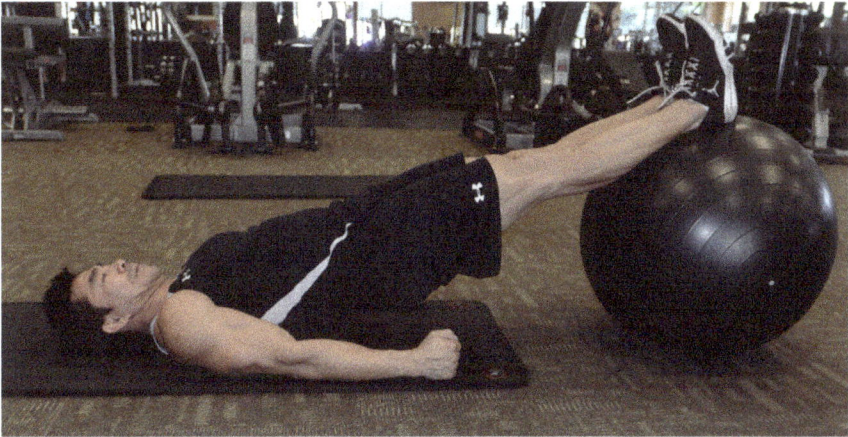

Core muscle exercises should be started from static positions and then progressed to dynamic exercises.

Exercise Each Muscle in Your Body

The Centers for Disease Control (CDC) recommends that muscle strengthening exercises for each major muscle group be done for two or more days per week. The major muscles can be easily divided into three simple groups: pushing, legs, and pulling. I recommend one day for each group with a rest day in between. Muscles grow during the rest/recovery periods.

Monday:	Pushing or chest, shoulders, triceps.
Tuesday:	Rest and/or cardio.
Wednesday:	Legs.
Thursday:	Rest and/or cardio.
Friday:	Pulling or back and biceps.
Saturday:	Rest/cardio.
Sunday:	Free—no exercise.

Begin each exercise day with five to ten minutes of cardiovascular exercise as a warmup. Next, perform foam roller release followed by active/dynamic stretching. Then perform one or two core exercises.

The first exercise for each major muscle group is a warmup exercise and is performed at 50%. Every fourth week, perform strength and stability exercises to strengthen the connective tissues. Stability exercises are performed while on an unstable surface, with the goal of activating stabilizers and trunk muscles.

Monday: Inclined 15-Degree Chest Press

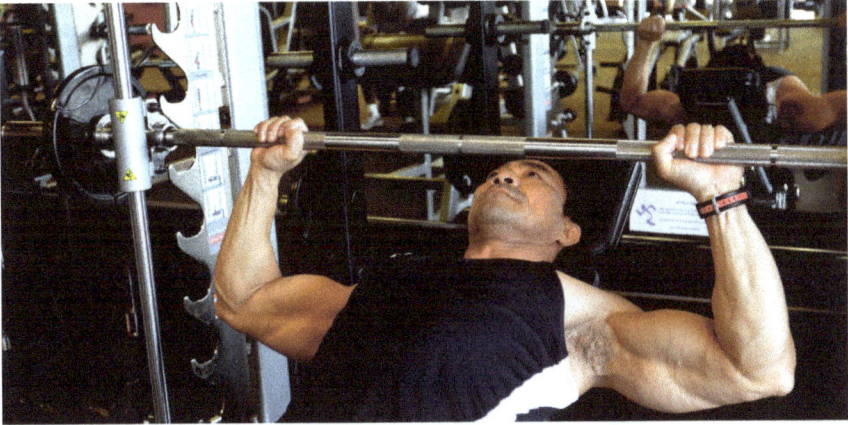

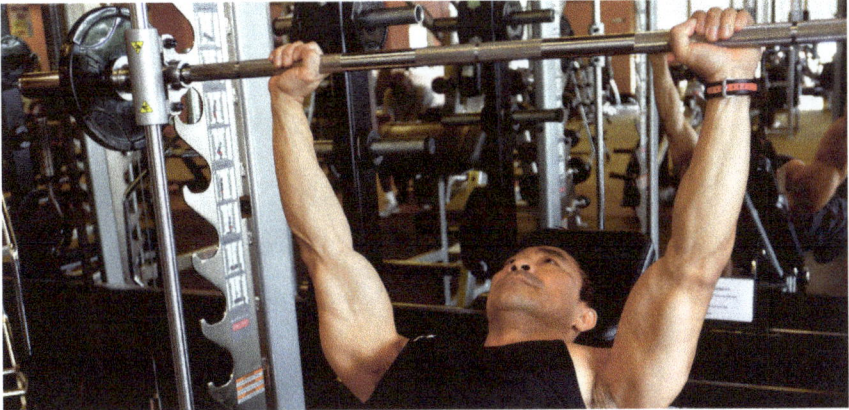

Monday: Seated Shoulder Press

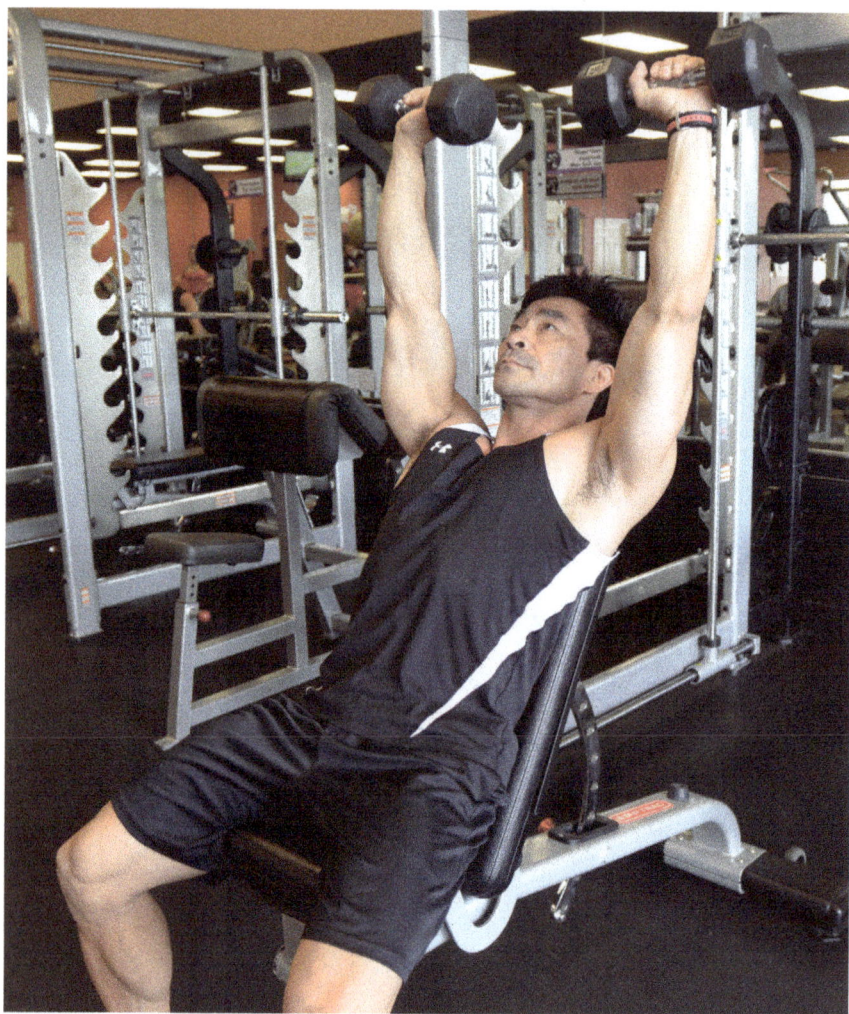

Monday: Seated Shoulder Press

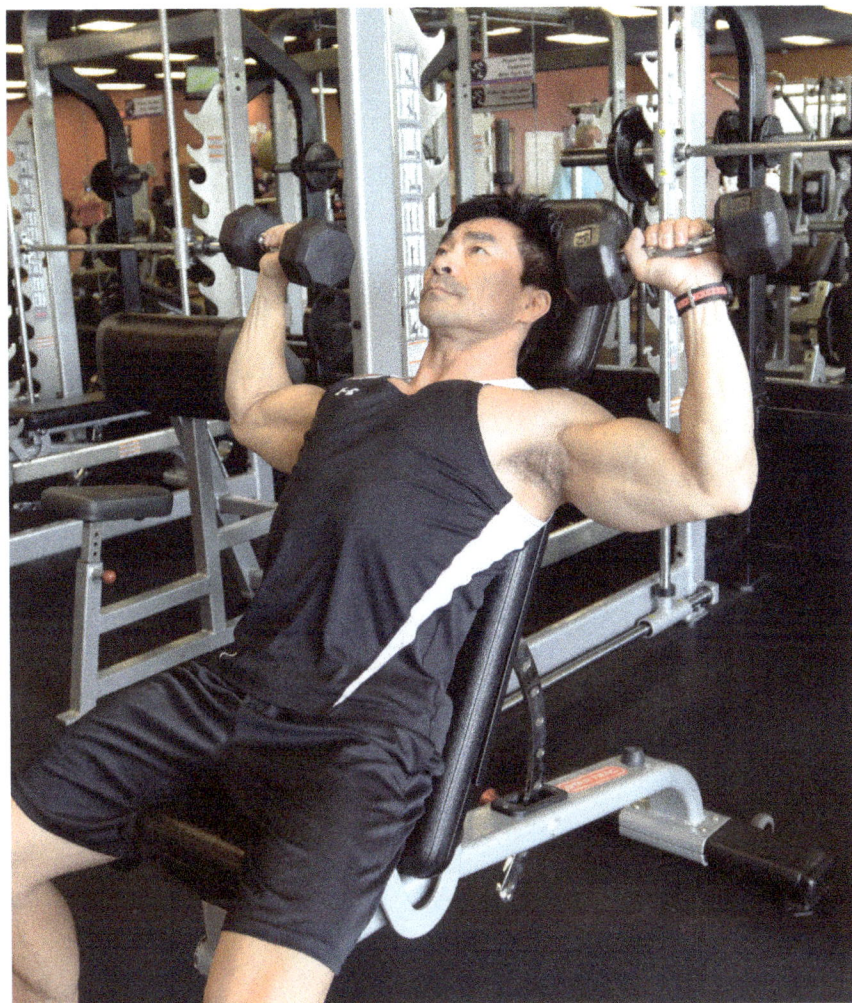

Monday: Triceps

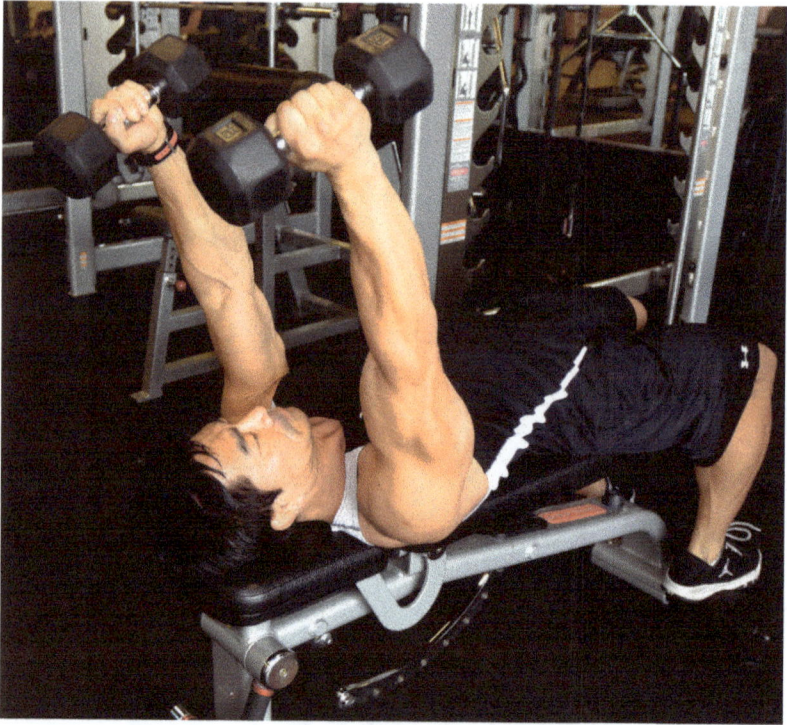

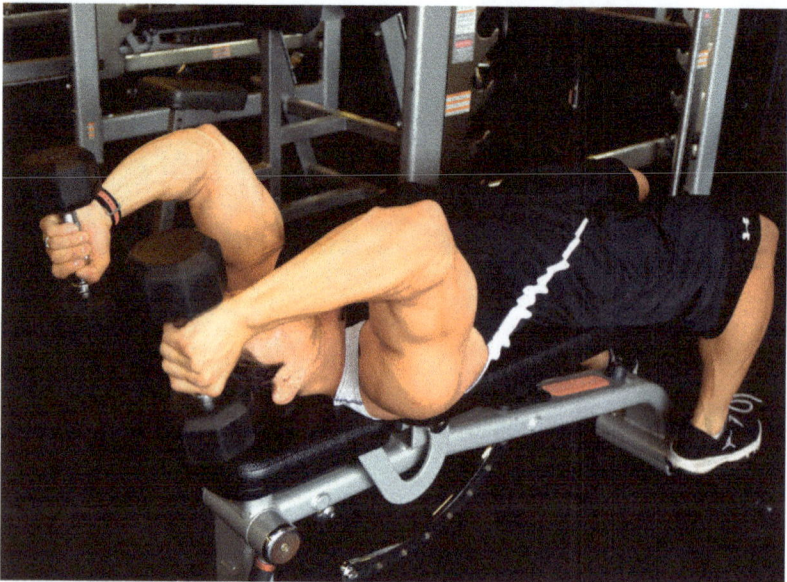

Wednesday: Leg Press

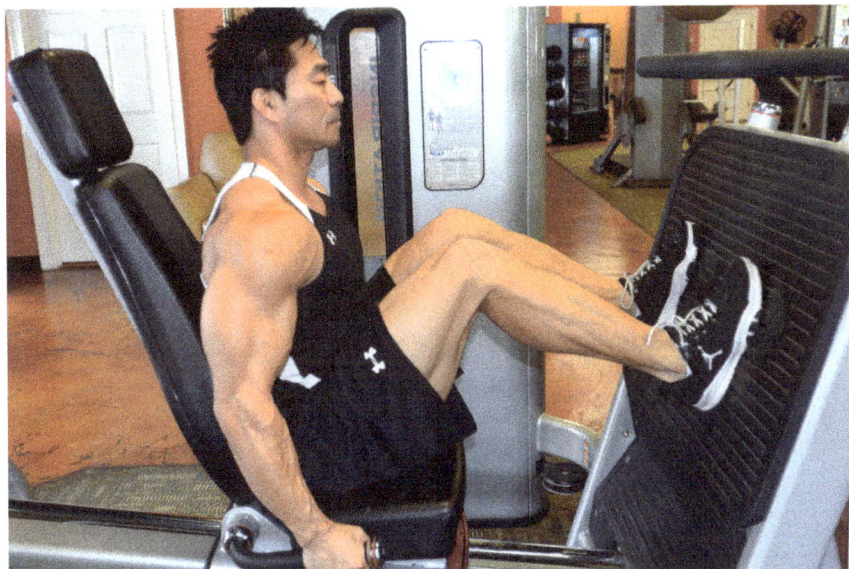

Wednesday: Leg Press

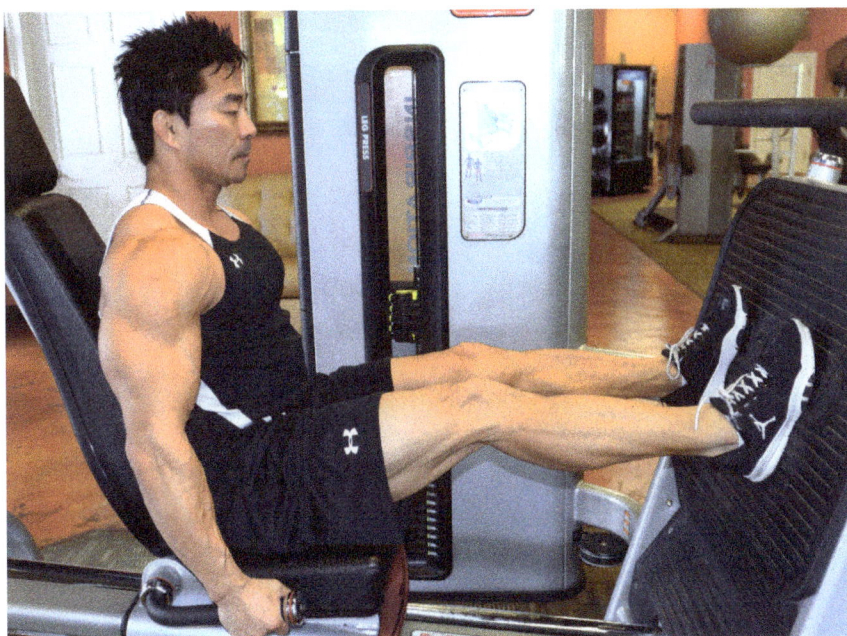

Wednesday: Legs—Smith Machine Squat

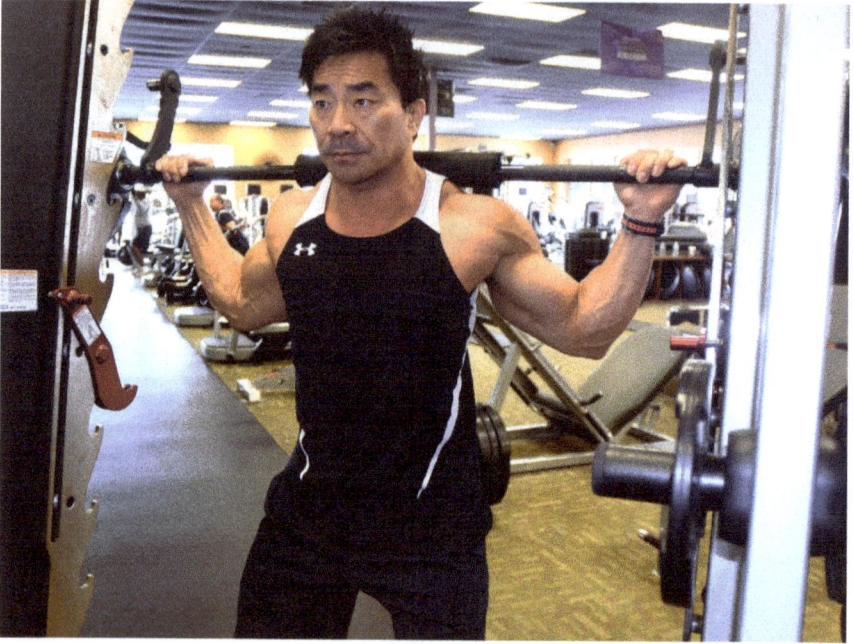

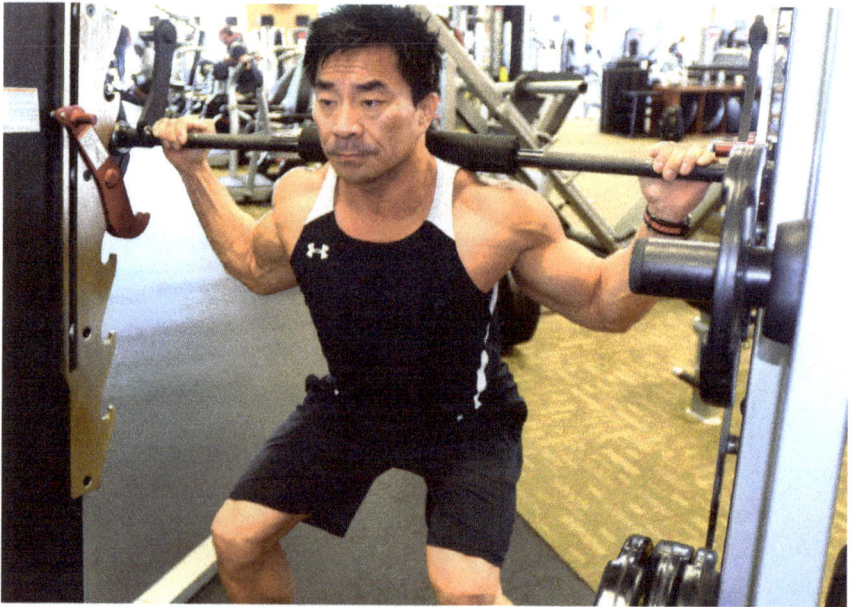

Wednesday: Leg Extensions

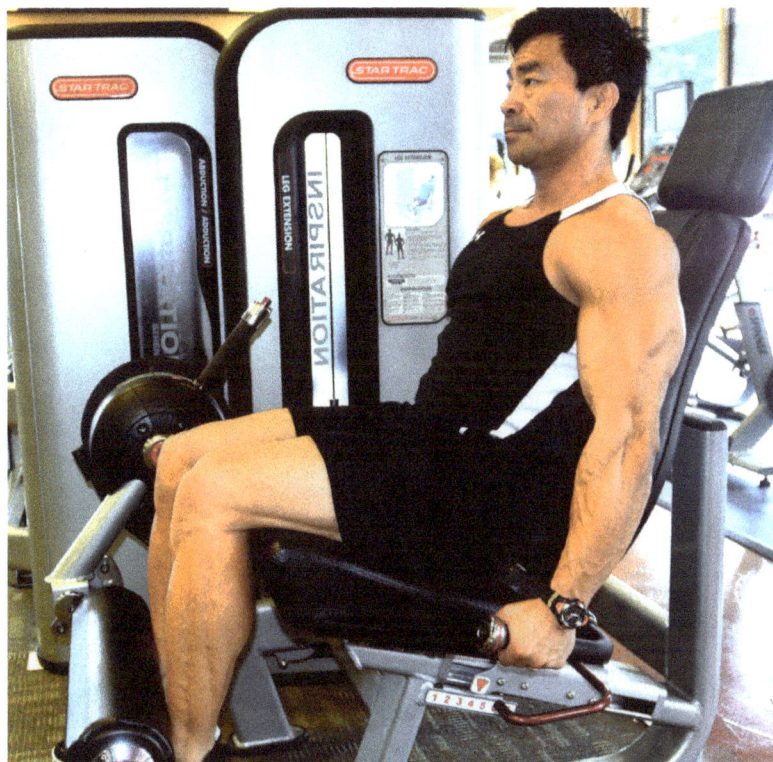

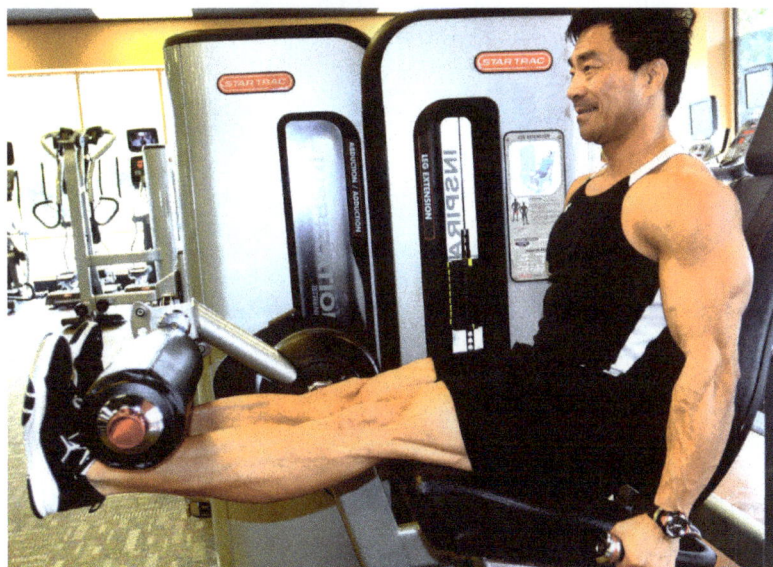

Wednesday: Legs—Hamstrings

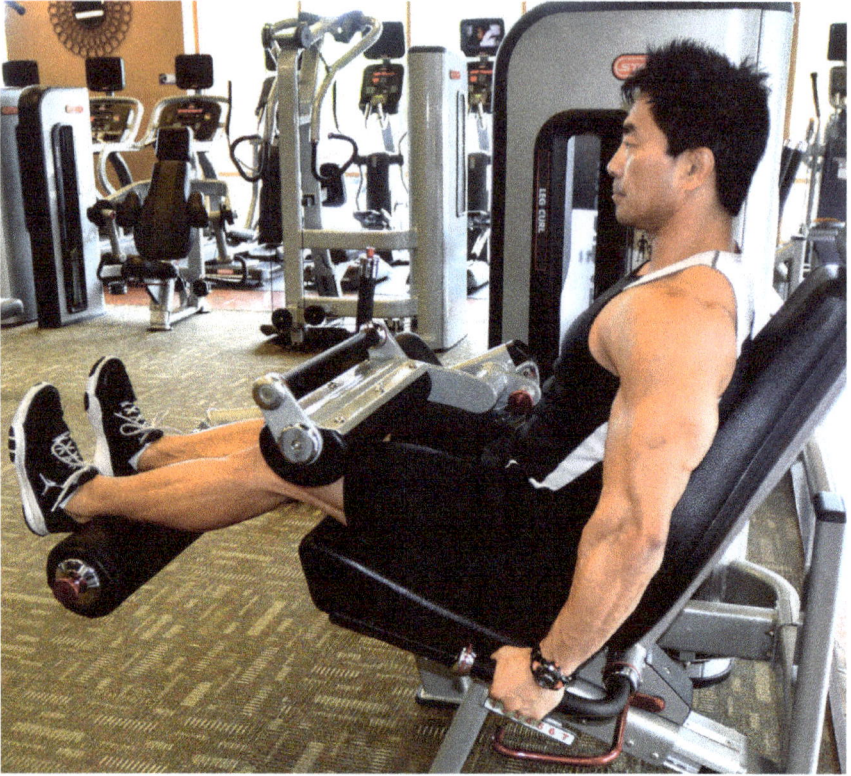

Wednesday: Legs—Hamstrings

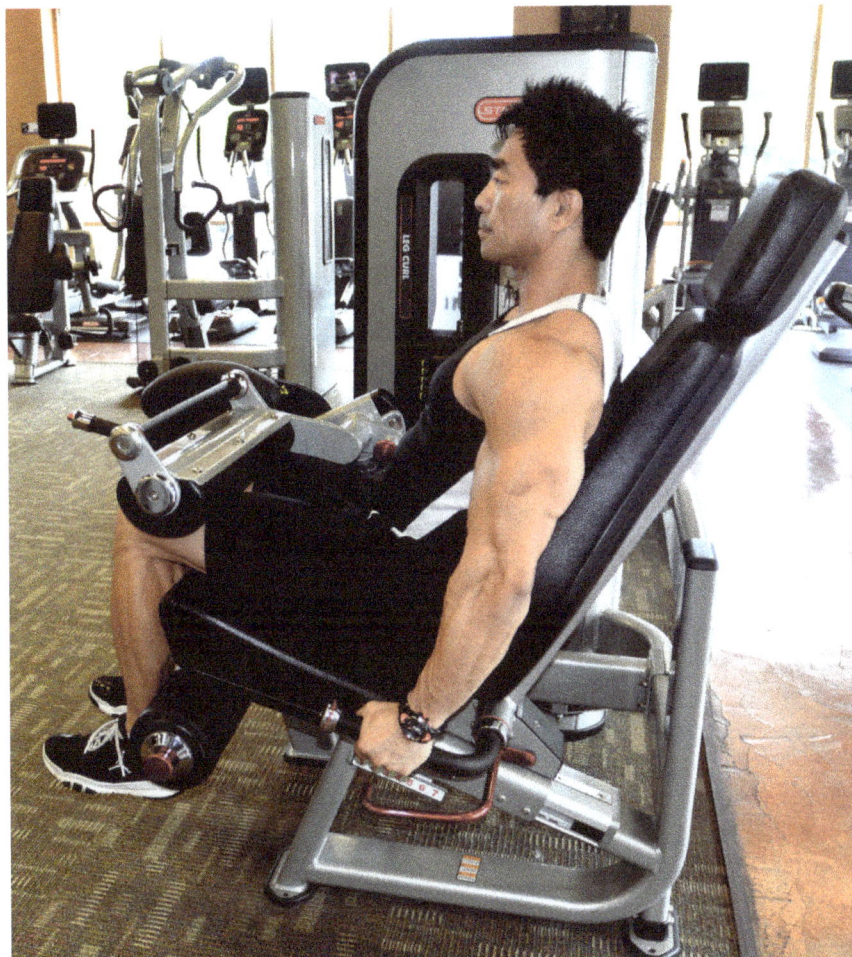

Friday: Back—Lat Pull-Down

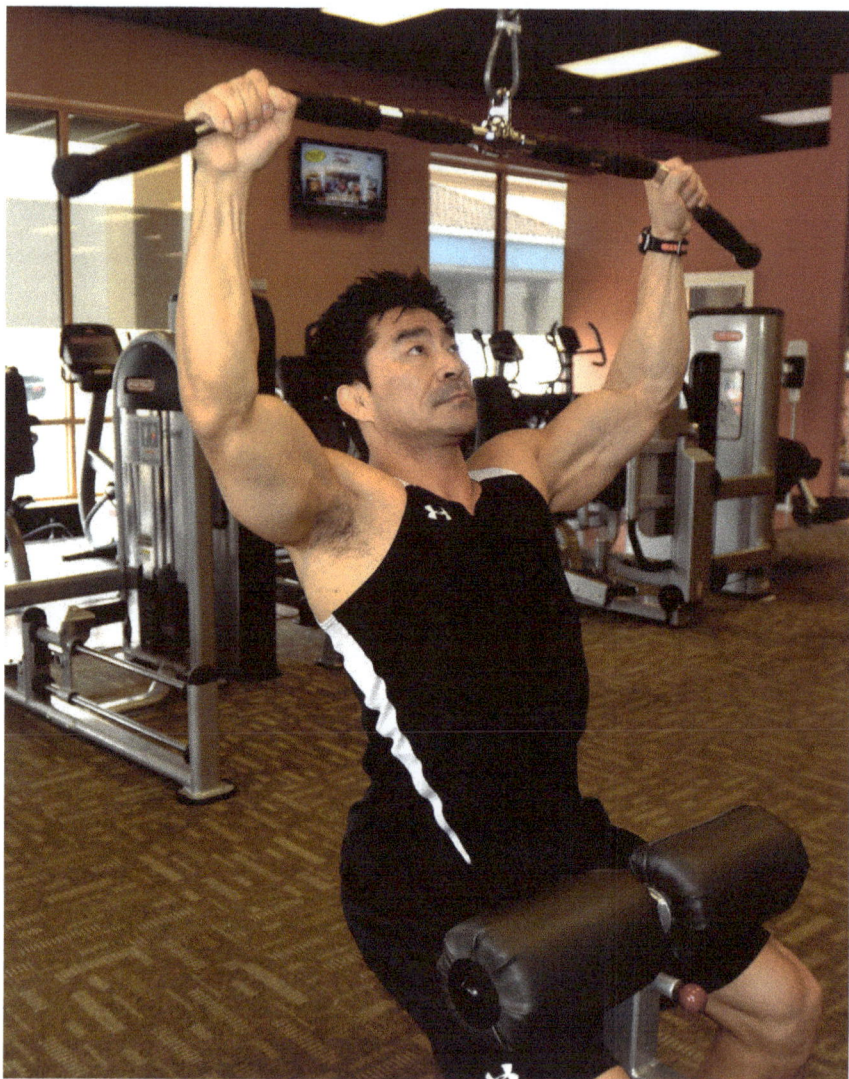

Friday: Back—Lat Pull-Down

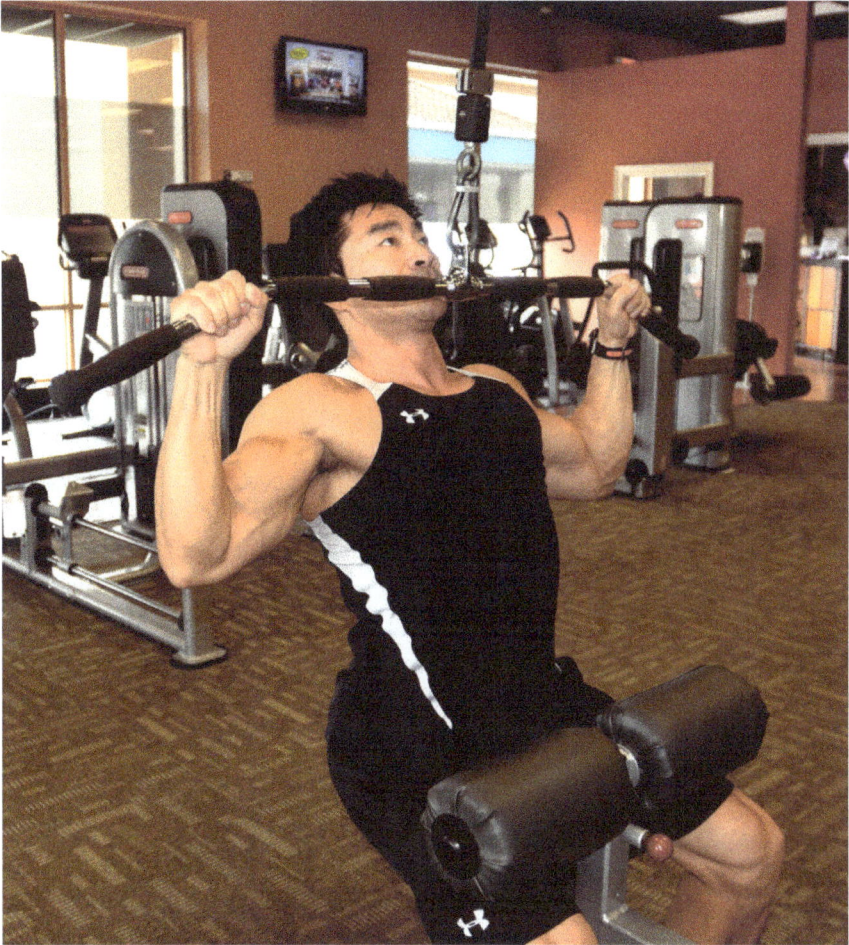

Friday: Back—Horizontal Row

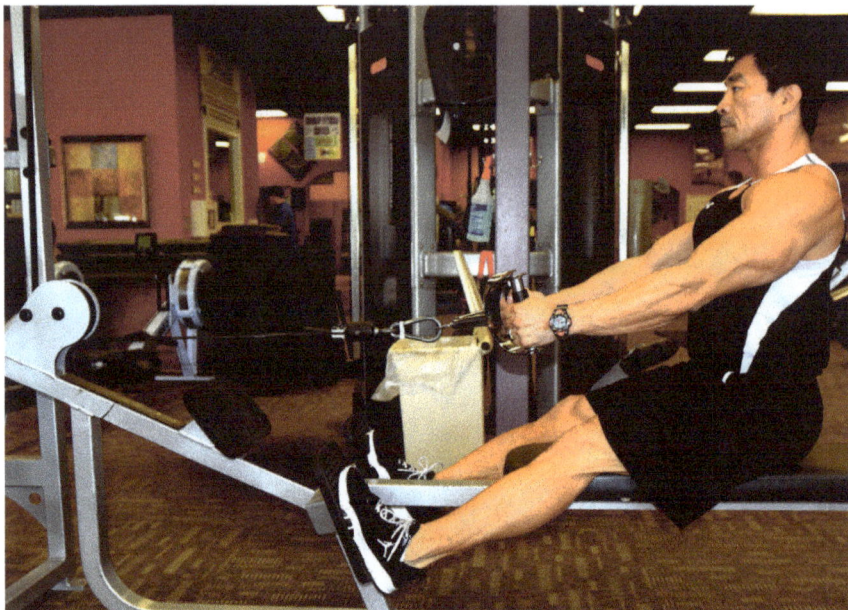

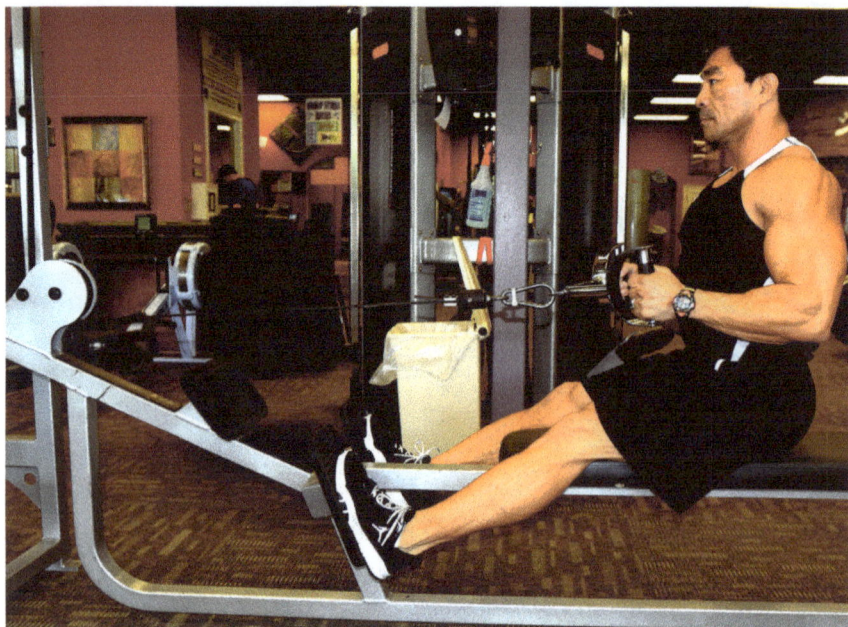

Friday: Biceps

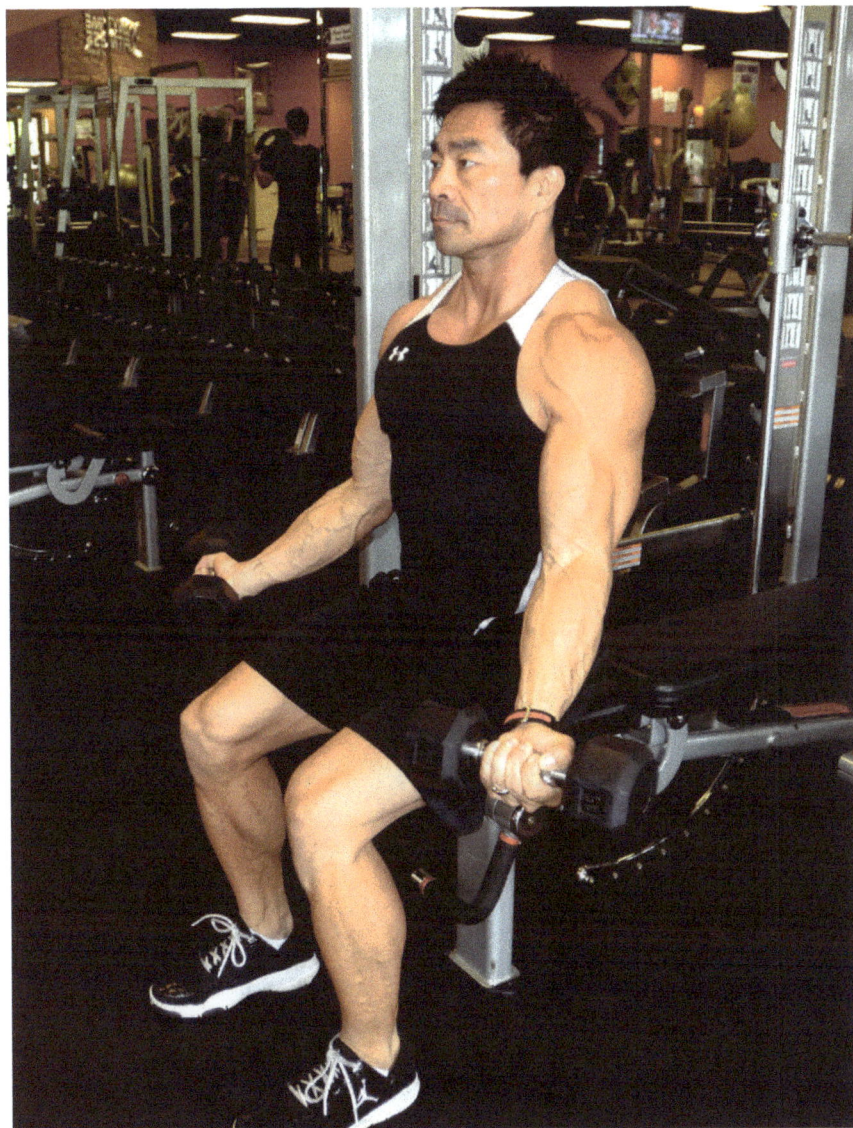

Friday: Biceps

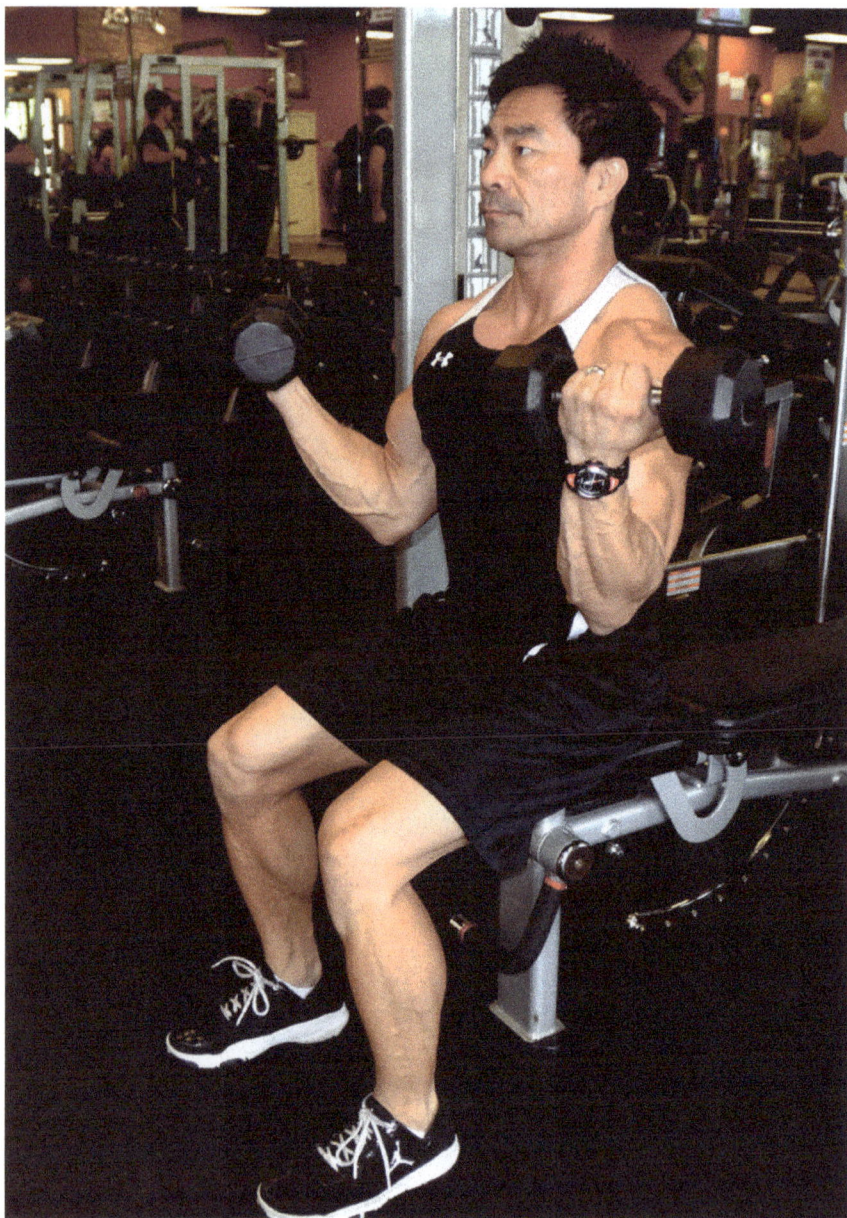

Monday & Friday: Abdominal Exercises

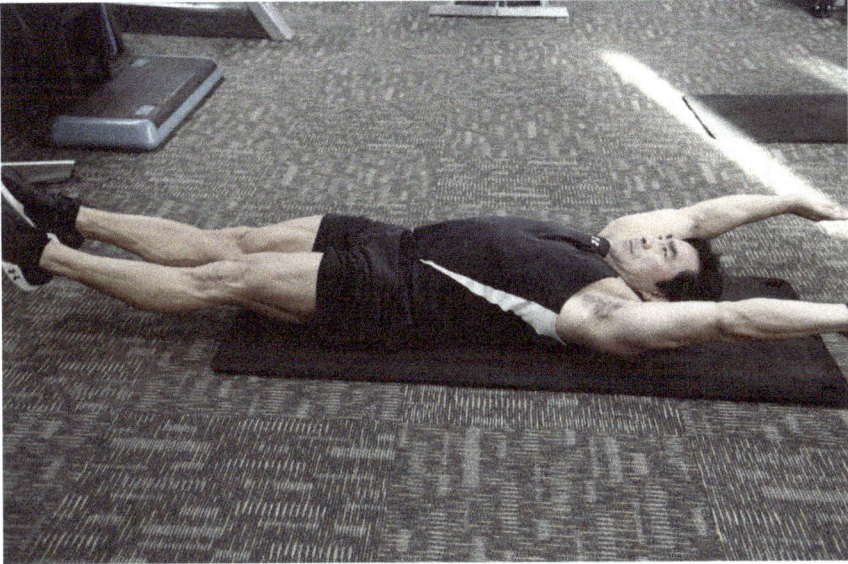

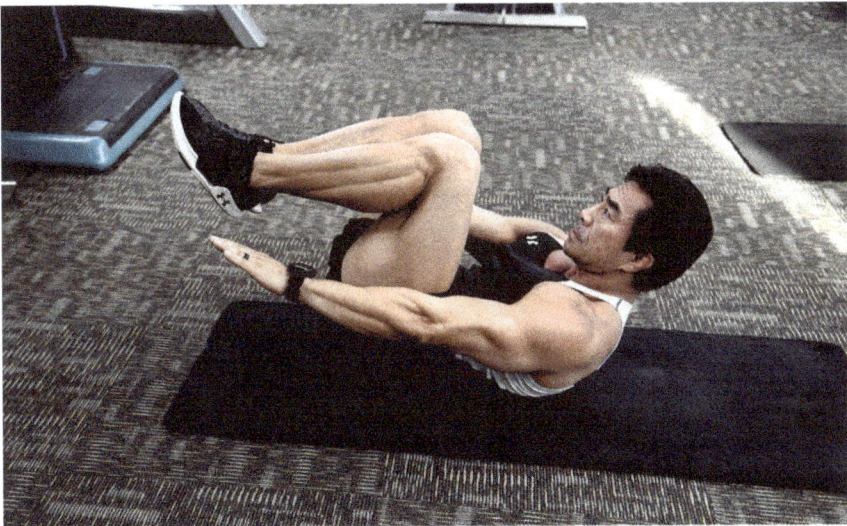

Abdominal muscles, like any other muscles, can be over-trained if exercised daily. These muscles need rest to grow; therefore, exercising two or three times a week is sufficient.

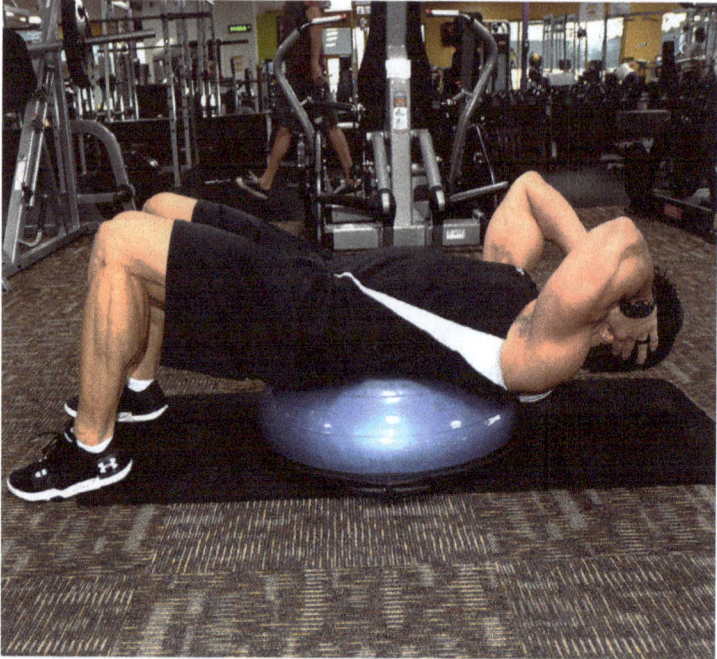

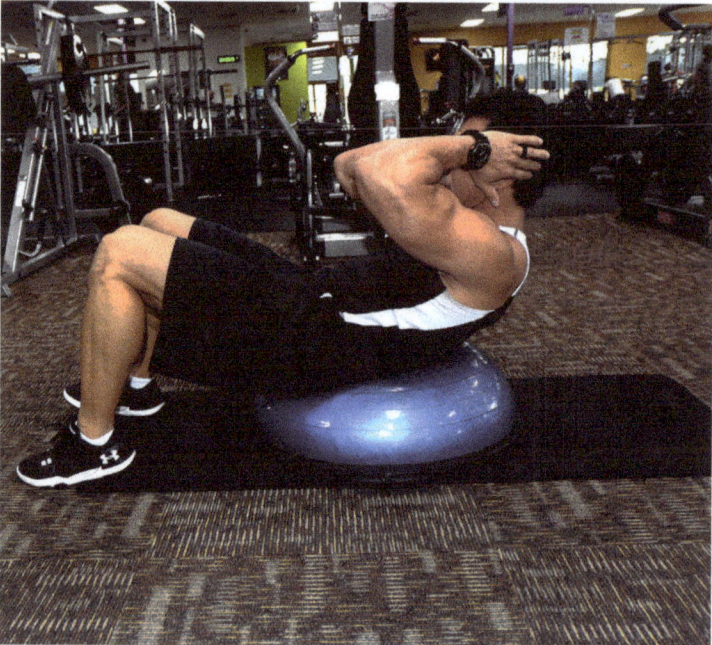

Core exercises that precede every workout also strengthen your abdominal muscles.

Being able to visibly see your abdominal muscles (six-pack abs) is more a question of your percentage of body fat than muscle bulk. You must be at or under 10% body fat in order to see your abdominal muscles. Thus, your diet is the key to having visible six-pack abs. Age and sex are not a factor—only body fat is. We all have abdominal muscles, but few of us are lean enough for them to be visible.

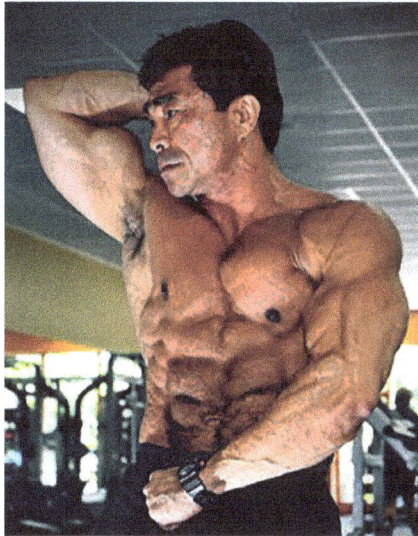

Six-Pack Abdominal Muscles
With 7% Body Fat

It will take a minimum of three months of resistance training, training to muscle failure three to four sessions per week, to realize an increase in strength [4]. It will take approximately three months to be able to visually observe changes.

You'll *feel* better within two weeks because you're using more muscles, improving insulin sensitivity, and raising testosterone levels. **Almost any physical activity will help to extend your life. Just 30 minutes of moderate activity four days a week or 20**

minutes of vigorous activity three times per week will increase one's life span by 27% in both men and women aged 50 to 70 years [5].

In addition to living longer, exercise helps to prevent disease. According to the American Heart Association, "Regular physical activity using large muscle groups, such as walking, running, or swimming, produces cardiovascular adaptations that increase exercise capacity, endurance, and skeletal muscle strength," [6]. Habitual physical activity also prevents the development of coronary artery disease (CAD) and reduces symptoms in patients with established cardiovascular disease. There is also evidence that exercise reduces the risk of other chronic diseases, including type 2 insulin-resistant diabetes, osteoporosis, obesity, depression, and cancer of the breast and colon.

Now you know that exercise is necessary, and you know how much exercising to do. What specific types of exercising should you do?

What Type of Exercise— Resistance or Endurance; Weights or Cardio?

The answer is that you need *both* resistance training and endurance training.

If you'd like to run a marathon, then cardiovascular training is most important; however, you'll still need to build strong leg muscles with some weight training. If, however, you want to compete in bodybuilding, then weight training for each muscle group is most important. However, you'll still need the benefits of endurance training—insulin sensitivity and cardiovascular health. Most people need both, and what predominates is a personal choice.

Weight or resistance exercise builds muscle mass and strength.

Cardiovascular exercise increases the use of oxygen in cells and leads to increased exercise capacity. If you decide to train for a serious endurance event, such as a marathon, you'll lose both body fat and muscle. This is because intense endurance exercises block the production of the muscle building enzyme mTOR [7].

In order to obtain the benefits of *both* resistance and cardiovascular exercise, you need to vary your routine *and* avoid doing both on the same day.

Heavy Weights With Few Repetitions? Light Weights With Frequent Repetitions?

The answer to this depends on your goal. If you desire to maintain muscle tone, *any* exercise to muscle failure will be sufficient as long as your diet is adequate.

In order to build or maintain muscle mass, you'll need adequate amino acids (protein), adequate carbohydrates to provide cellular energy, and adequate fats to ensure normal hormone levels.

If you're dieting and have a calorie deficit, then high resistance repetitions may cause muscle loss because endurance training with caloric restriction has been shown to decrease the enzymes required for muscle building and repair (the mTOR pathway) [8].

If you want to build muscle, you have to continuously overload your muscles with heavy weights and increase muscle protein synthesis while providing all the nutrients and hormones your body needs, including adequate protein, carbohydrates, and fat.

Can Exercise be Harmful?

Strenuous exercise can cause menstrual disorders in women [9]. In this study, 28 exercise-naïve women were asked to run four to 10 miles per day for two menstrual cycles and to engage in 3.5 hours of exercise every day. Only four of the 28 subjects had a normal menstrual cycle during these intense exercises. Thus, it was found that intense exercise can disturb reproductive function in women.

Long-term training for, and competing in, extreme endurance events—such as marathons and ironman distance triathlons—can cause transient acute volume overload of the right heart (atria and ventricle), leading to damage of the heart muscle and the development of cardiac arrhythmias [10].

A common problem found in endurance athletes is lower-extremity stress fractures [11]. A stress fracture occurs when muscles become fatigued and are unable to absorb additional force. In time, fatigued muscle transfers the overload to the bone, causing a tiny crack (stress fracture) in the bone. Stress fractures of the lower extremities are common injuries among individuals who participate in high load-bearing endurance activities, such as long-distance running. Stress fracture incidence in runners approaches 16% of all injuries.

Perhaps the most dangerous complication of excessive exercise and dehydration is rhabdomyolysis. Rhabdomyolysis is the rapid death of muscle cells and the subsequent release of a dangerous protein (myoglobin) into the bloodstream, which can cause kidney damage and elevation of serum potassium that can adversely, possibly even fatally, affect the heart.

Schiff et al. studied 44 runners who completed a 99-km road race and found that 25 of the runners demonstrated increased blood levels of myoglobin. Myoglobin was detected in the post-race urine samples of only six runners. Acute renal failure was not observed in any of these subjects. In another study, 24 athletes who had competed in a triathlon showed a dramatic rise in serum myoglobin and reported muscle pain, but none required hospitalization [12].

Knee injuries are very common. This is usually caused by weak muscles in the legs, weak core muscles, and misalignment of the knees in relation to the feet.

Shoulder muscles are also easily injured because the shoulder joint is not designed for weight bearing and is made from the confluence of soft tissues. Preventing shoulder injuries requires strict adherence to form and technique. The muscles and tendons surrounding the shoulder joint keep the head of the upper arm bone firmly in the rotator cuff (the shallow socket of the shoulder). Any injury to these soft tissues can cause the upper arm bone to strike or impinge on the shoulder bone, causing pain.

Muscles weakened from years of disuse are easily injured. If pain occurs during a leg or shoulder exercise, it's best to immediately stop the exercise, rest and ice the muscle, apply a compression garment, and elevate the extremity if possible. If pain persists, you may need to visit your physician.

Intense exercise requires a recovery period. Inadequate recovery and continued exercise stress leads to tissue damage.

Lower back injuries are common when first beginning an exercise routine. The core muscles connect the chest to the pelvis. Weak core muscles cannot maintain proper spinal alignment, resulting in lower back pain and injury. Back injuries can be prevented with proper warmup exercises and strong core muscles. When exercising, you should always schedule rest days in between weight-training days.

Treatment of most lower back pain includes rest, over-the-counter anti-inflammatory medications such as ibuprofen, massage therapy, acupuncture, and chiropractic treatments. Core muscle strength is the best protection against lower back injury.

If pain persists and prevents routine daily activity, then you need to see your doctor. Surgery is always the last resort.

Vibration Therapy

The history of vibration therapy to improve athletic performance started in 1857 with Dr. Gustav Zander. Initially, machines were developed for whole-body vibration. In the 1990s, Russian scientists used vibration therapy to successfully repair the muscle loss and the bone density loss of returning astronauts. Whole-body vibration requires you to position yourself on a machine with a vibrating platform. This forces your muscles to contract and relax dozens of times each second. Many people claim that this treatment provides the same benefits as exercise. There are no prospective randomized studies of whole-body vibration therapy—thus, only level 3 to 4 data. Localized vibration therapy has recently become available and appears to have significant clinical benefits in controlled clinical trials [13, 14]. Localized vibration therapy increases blood flow and decreases pain in the area treated [15]. Localized vibration therapy has become a popular home therapy option for athletes using the commercially available TheraGun. According to the TheraGun Company, their device **will reduce muscle pain, decrease the time of rehabilitation for muscle injuries, increase blood flow to injured tissues, increase lymphatic flow, and provide rapid myofascial release both pre workout and post workout.**

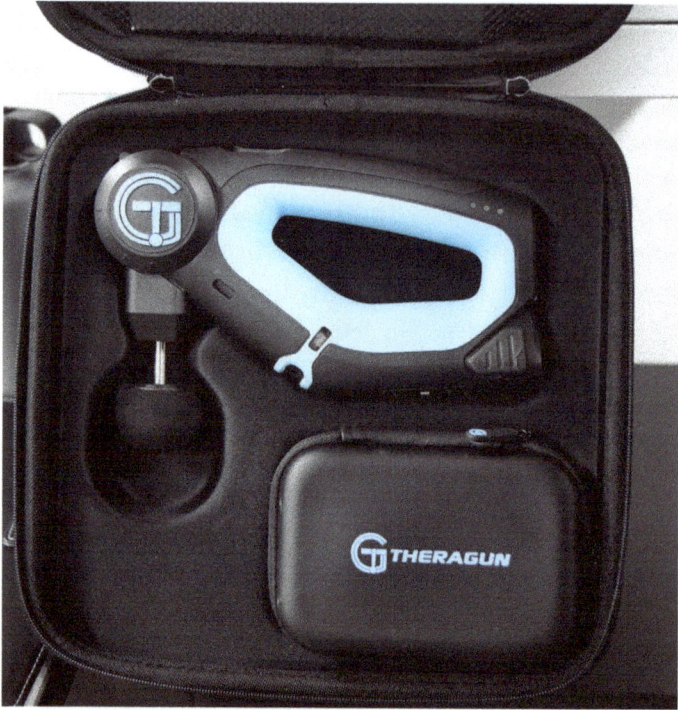

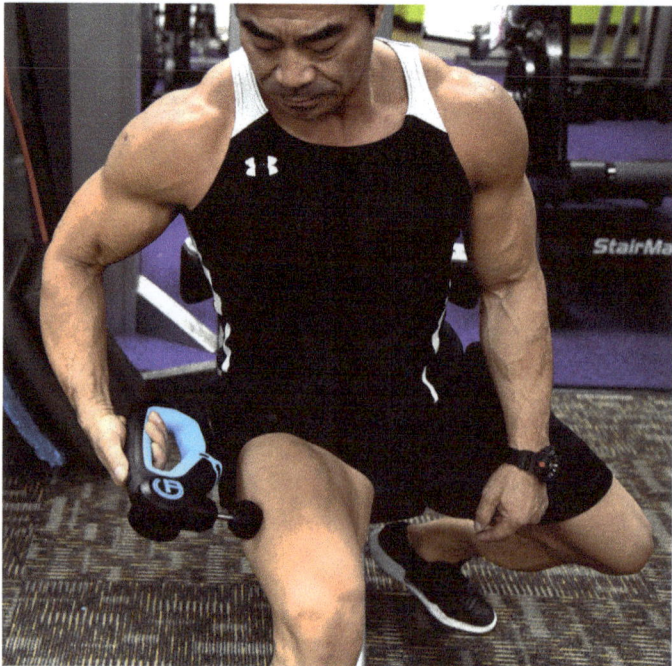

How to Choose a Personal Trainer

If you can afford a personal trainer, do it. Even if your lessons are few and all you learn is how to use gym equipment, your body will benefit.

Finding a good trainer isn't easy. Your trainer must be certified by an established organization, such as the American Council on Exercise (ACE), National Academy of Sports Medicine (NASM), International Sports Science Association (ISSA), American College of Sports Medicine (ACSM), or National Strength and Conditioning Association (NSCA). It's ideal if your trainer has had additional post-certification training in human muscle kinetics.

You can tell a good trainer from a bad one by making a few simple observations. Your trainer should focus entirely upon you during your session and not be conversing with other people. He or she should answer your questions with ease.

Your trainer should evaluate your abilities, ask you for your goals, and provide a road map so you can attain those goals. If your trainer doesn't guide you through dynamic stretching, you have the wrong trainer. A good trainer will integrate a corrective strategy into your program and help to prevent injuries while you pursue your fitness goals.

Your trainer should evaluate your current posture and joint move-ment—the musculoskeletal dysfunction that you're bringing into the gym from your current lifestyle. What you bring into the gym may cause injuries in the future, and these need to be prevented.

Two simple observations: your posture, both standing still and when sitting, reveals important information. Your trainer should look for the three common patterns of dysfunction: flat feet and knock-knees; forward pelvic tilt; and rounded shoulders with head forward [16].

Posture, Standing Still:
Flat Feet & Knock-Knees

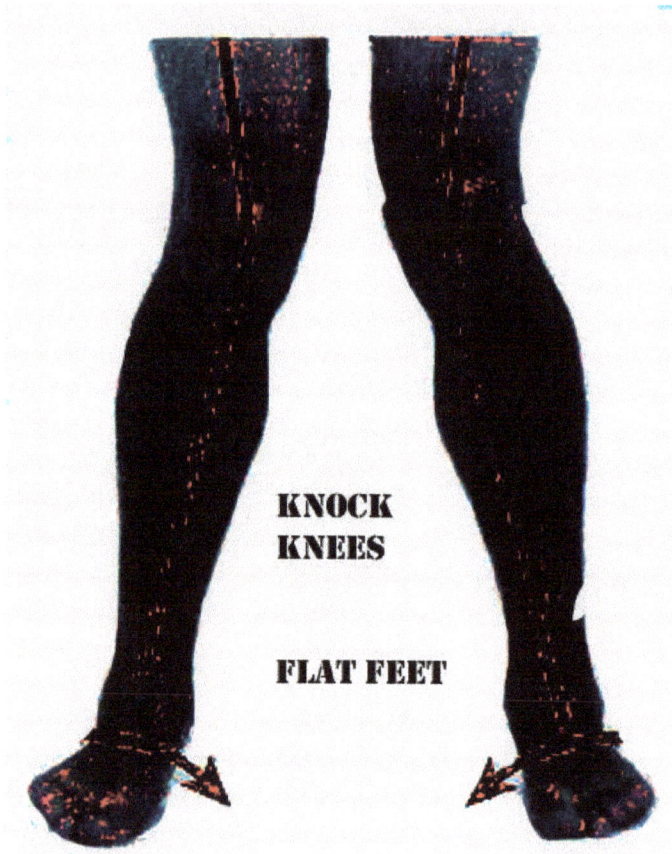

KNOCK
KNEES

FLAT FEET

This dysfunction can lead to foot pain, shin splints, knee pain, and lower back pain.

Forward Pelvic Tilt

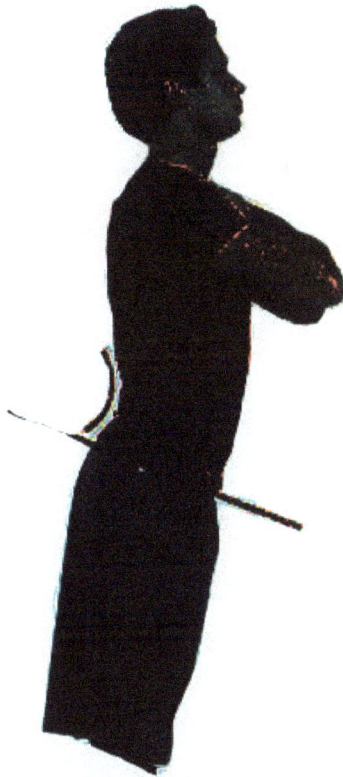

FORWARD PELVIC TILT

This dysfunction leads to hamstring (three posterior upper thigh muscles) injuries and pain, knee pain, and lower back pain.

Rounded Shoulders & Forward Head

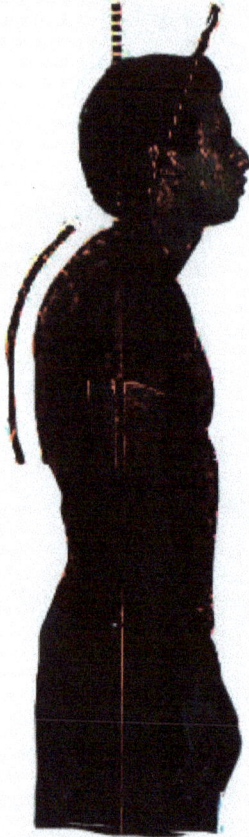

ROUNDED SHOULDERS AND FORWARD HEAD TILT

This dysfunction leads to headaches, bicep tendonitis, shoulder (rotator cuff) pain, and numbness and pain in the neck, hands, and fingers.

Your posture when sitting (dynamic posture) will provide additional information regarding muscle strength or weakness, balance, and joint movement.

Dynamic Posture Assessment

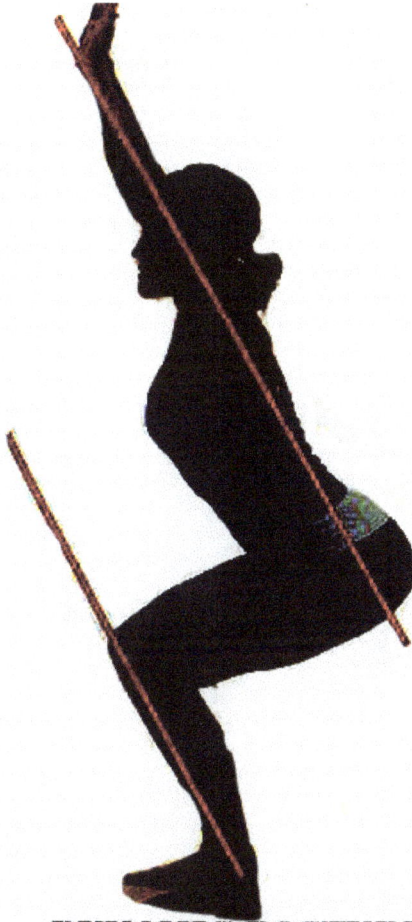

DYNAMIC POSTURE

Dynamic and static posture evaluations will provide information which allows your trainer to select the appropriate training exercises to correct your specific weaknesses. There are many dynamic exercises available.

Master Trainer Donny Kim, PES, CPT-NASM

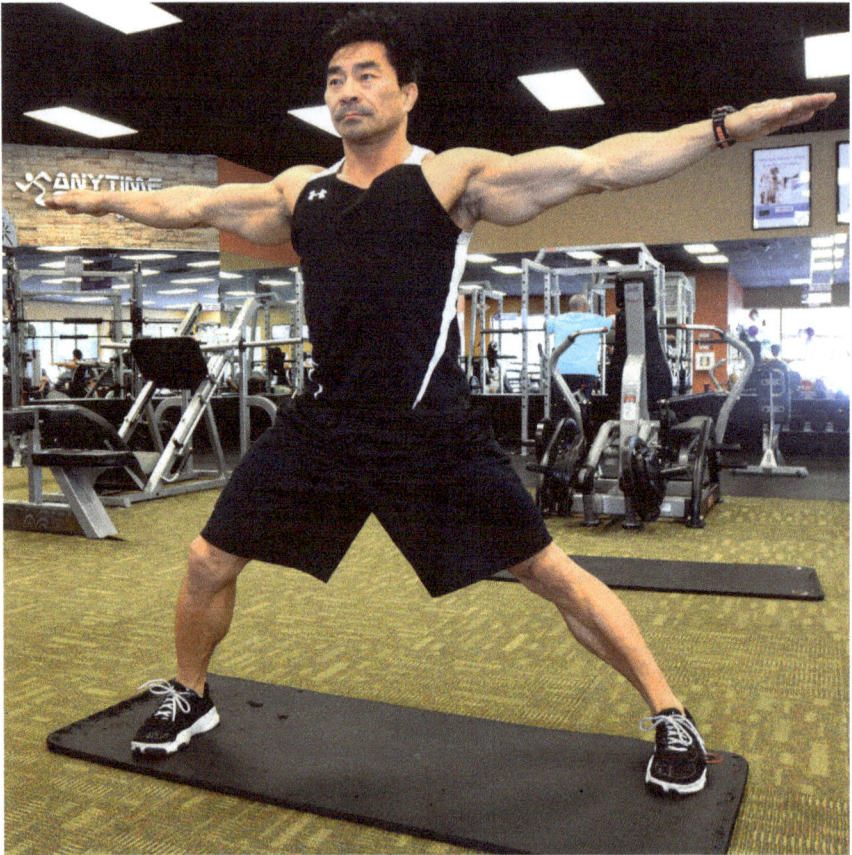

CHAPTER 15
The Holy Grail: How to Lose Fat and Build Muscle at the Same Time

With athletes who are involved in resistance training and dieting to lose body fat, **the speed of weight loss is the important factor in the preservation of muscle mass [1].**

Losing approximately one pound per week or precisely 0.7% of your body weight per week may be ideal. It's possible to increase lean body mass by 0.2% with this slow regimen of dieting and strength training.

Loss of approximately two pounds per week or 1.7% of your body weight per week causes no gain or slight loss of lean body mass.

The place to start your diet, as previously mentioned, is to first calculate how many calories per day you need in order to maintain your current weight. Then take this number and subtract 500 calories; this is your caloric starting point. This number will now be converted into proteins per day, carbohydrates per day, and fats per day.

The next calculation involves calories devoted to protein. The minimum protein intake for active athletes is 1.4 grams of protein intake for every 2.203 pounds of body weight. A diet higher in protein, such as 25% to 40% of total calories, will decrease appetite and increase satiety. In simple terms, you won't be hungry, and you'll eat less.

High-protein diets produce a sustained decrease in ad lib caloric intake that may be mediated by increased central nervous system leptin sensitivity and results in significant weight loss. This anorexic effect of protein may contribute to the weight loss produced by low-carbohydrate diets [2]. Dieting athletes require a relatively high protein intake to minimize loss of lean body mass.

As mentioned earlier, fat accompanies protein sources and may be equally responsible for the benefits of this high-protein, high-fat diet. Assuming you exercise, the minimum fat content in your diet should be 30% to 40% of all calories, and protein 30% to 40%. The remaining calories in your diet are for intermediate glycemic carbohydrates. The caloric content of low glycemic carbohydrates such as green vegetables and salads do not count because the energy required to metabolize them equals their calorie content. Intermediate glycemic carbohydrates such as yams and oatmeal are needed if you wish to build muscle.

A refeed consists of a brief overfeeding period during which caloric intake is raised slightly above maintenance levels, wherein the increase in caloric intake is predominantly achieved by increasing carbohydrate consumption. Athletes such as bodybuilders and figure competitors may abandon their strict diets one day each week as needed and rebuild the glycogen stores of the liver.

The proposed goal of this periodic refeeding is to temporarily increase circulating leptin, lower ghrelin, and stimulate the metabolic rate. There is evidence indicating that leptin is acutely responsive to short-term overfeeding [4].

Caffeine or coffee will help one lose body fat—see the section on supplements.

Fat Loss—Muscle Gain—The Holy Grail

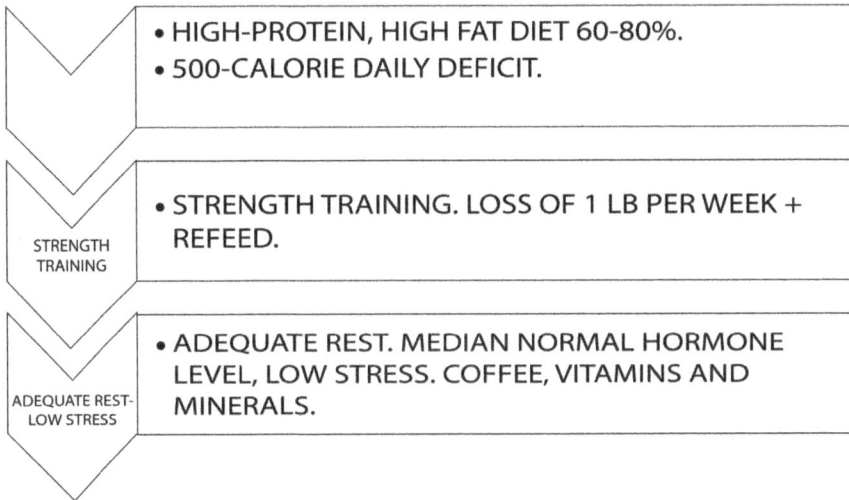

- HIGH-PROTEIN, HIGH FAT DIET 60-80%.
- 500-CALORIE DAILY DEFICIT.

STRENGTH TRAINING
- STRENGTH TRAINING. LOSS OF 1 LB PER WEEK + REFEED.

ADEQUATE REST- LOW STRESS
- ADEQUATE REST. MEDIAN NORMAL HORMONE LEVEL, LOW STRESS. COFFEE, VITAMINS AND MINERALS.

In order to build muscle tissue, your sex hormone levels and thyroid hormone levels *must* be in the median normal range, preferably in the upper ranges of normal. This is essential.

Example of My Fat Loss Holy Grail Diet

My basal resting calories are approximately 2000 calories per day, so 2000 – 500 = 1,500 calories to lose approximately one pound per week or less.

BREAKFAST, MEAL 1: 5:00 a.m.—½ cup Quaker old-fashioned oatmeal made with water, 1 protein shake, 3 boiled eggs and my supplements (multivitamins, calcium, Vitamin D3, krill oil, creatine, HMB (beta-hydroxy beta-methylbutyric acid), CoQ10, and minerals) = 600 calories. Total 44 grams of protein, 40 grams of carbohydrate, 32 grams of fat.

MEAL 2: 9:00 a.m.—5 ounces of chicken breast, 1 cup sweet potato and salad = 390 calories. 27 grams of protein, 13 grams of fat, 55 grams of carbohydrate.

MEAL 3: noon to 1:00 p.m.—4 ounces of chicken leg or thigh, and salad = 150 calories, 22 grams of protein, and 7 grams of fat.

MEAL 4: 6–7 p.m.—6 ounces of grilled salmon and salad.

MEAL 5: 9–10 p.m.—light protein shake of 100 calories, 20 grams of protein, 2 grams of fat, 3 grams of carbohydrate.

Total calories = 1510; 137 grams of protein (36%); 74 grams of fat (44%) and approximately 40 grams of intermediate glycemic carbohydrates (20%), not counting the salad carbohydrates. These are approximate values. I exercise in the morning and have the majority of my carbohydrates earlier in the day.

Weight training as usual—each muscle group to complete failure—Monday: pushing exercises; Wednesday: legs; Friday: pulling exercises. Cardiovascular exercises for 30 to 40 minutes each evening. If I wake up hungry between midnight and 3:00 a.m., I'll add a protein shake to help me return to sleep.

In summary, the goal of this diet is to lose slightly less or equal to one pound of body fat per week while building muscle. This will give you an approximate starting place; you'll find that things change over time, and you'll need to adjust in order to succeed. Keep a written or digital (such as in your cell phone) journal every day, and keep the faith!

Carbohydrate Cycling—Extreme

Carbohydrate cycling is controversial and may not be needed by most athletes. There have been no prospective or randomized studies proving the benefit of carbohydrate cycling. If it works for you, then it's good.

The idea is similar to the concept of refeeding. You will lose body fat quickly on a low-carb diet, as outlined above. Leptin decreases, your brain lowers the metabolic rate, and muscle synthesis decreases due to the lack of glycogen stores (low cellular energy) [4].

Fat loss plateaus as your body seeks to remain constant (homeostasis). When you increase carbohydrate intake, leptin levels increase as fat cells are replenished, and you'll be able to build muscle with a greater source of cellular energy from glycogen.

The purpose of cycling carbohydrates is to benefit from both fat loss and muscle gain **by eating more carbohydrates on days of strenuous exercise and decreasing carbohydrates on days of rest or less strenuous exercise.**

A typical carbohydrate cycle might look like this:

Day 1:   100-200 grams carbs (400-800 calories)—chest/pushing exercises.

Day 2:   30-50 grams carbs (120-200 calories)—rest or 30 minutes cardio.

Day 3:   100-200 grams carbs (400-800 calories)—leg exercises.

Day 4:   30-50 grams carbs (120-200 calories)—rest or 30 minutes cardio.

Day 5:   100-200 grams carbs (400-800 calories)—back/pulling exercises.

Days 6&7: Variable, depending on results.

It's important to adjust your carbohydrate intake to meet your goals. A daily diary of your body measurements is helpful. Carbohydrate cycling may benefit most athletes trying to lose body fat, whose body fat is already below 10%—these are extreme bodybuilders.

The best sources of carbohydrates are oatmeal, grits, yams, and brown rice. Fibrous carbohydrates, such as salads and most vegetables, can be eaten freely without measure. Avoid wheat products and most dairy except Greek yogurt. Wheat contains gluten, which can cause digestive inflammation, and dairy products produce excessive insulin—more than their sugar content owing to stimulation of glucagon-like peptide 1.

"I Joined a Gym, I Exercise, and I Look the Same"—Anthony's Story

Anthony is the 48-year-old owner of a software company. He's been going to the gym three days a week and lifting weights with his friends. He states that he eats a healthy diet and doesn't eat desserts or fried foods.

Anthony complains that his body image hasn't changed in two years—in fact, he's been gaining weight and has been unable to lose his love handles (abdominal fat overhanging his pants), as well as being unable to see the six-pack abs that he had in high school.

When he was in high school, he weighed 150 pounds, and now, 30 years later, he weighs 185 pounds with a BMI of 28.

His blood work showed normal kidney and liver function, low free and total testosterone, normal estradiol, normal HGB-A1C, elevated triglycerides, slightly elevated LDL, and slightly low HDL. His blood pressure was elevated at 150/90. His waist-to-height ratio was 0.58.

His physical exam was normal with no visible or palpable evidence of disease. A review of his family history indicated that his father developed coronary heart disease at age 66.

With a BMI above 25, Anthony is overweight. He hasn't yet developed any measurable metabolic damage, but with hypertension, abnormal lipids and excess visceral body fat based upon his waist-to-height ratio > 0.5, he is at increased risk for future cardiovascular disease.

Like many, Anthony didn't calculate his caloric intake. Using a daily food diary, I calculated that he'd been consuming approximately 3,000 calories per day—a caloric excess of approximately 400 calories per day.

The exercises he'd been doing at the gym were high repetitions with light weights, and his gym days were more of a social meeting with friends than anything else. He did 60 minutes of light cardiovascular exercise on a treadmill before lifting weights. He actually only visited the gym twice a week and rarely, if ever, exercised his legs; and he *never* exercised his core muscles.

Anthony was making many mistakes.

1. He was consuming too many calories, so his body was making and storing body fat. In order to lose body fat, he requires a maximum of 2,100 calories per day (a 500-calorie deficit against his caloric maintenance level). He should aim to lose one pound per week.

2. His cardiovascular exercise was ineffective; it didn't incorporate high-intensity interval training (HIIT).

3. Doing cardiovascular exercise *before* resistance or weight training shuts down the metabolic pathways to building muscle.

4. Weight training to build muscle must include heavy weights to continuously and progressively stress the muscle. More muscle increases metabolic rate and energy output.

5. Your legs have the biggest muscles in your body and

provide a strong base, along with the core muscles, which allows you to increase upper-body muscle strength by using heavier weights. If your core and leg muscles are weak, you can't lift heavier weights; this limits your ability to build new muscle.

6. Anthony's total and free testosterone levels were low, and he did not wish to start hormone replacement therapy at first.

Anthony encountered much difficulty in changing his diet and lifestyle. Upon initiation of hormone replacement therapy to obtain median normal levels, Anthony has started to show improvement in muscle development and energy levels.

CHAPTER 16
What is a Dietary Supplement?

Dietary supplements provide substances that may be needed but are missing from your diet. Supplements are not intended to treat disease; they're intended to ensure peak performance by adding something that may be missing from the foods you're eating. The most widely used supplements in the U.S. are multivitamins [1].

One reason you may need supplements is that with vigorous exercise, your body needs time to recover, repair itself, and build new muscle. Supplements may help your body to recover and prevent injuries, especially if you are decreasing your calorie/ food intake and increasing your exercise. **As an athlete, you are different from the average American, and you have different needs.**

Most supplements are not needed if you don't regularly do vigorous exercise, since a balanced diet can provide all essential nutrients. If you're eating a high-protein diet and are **exercising vigorously, you shouldn't consider yourself to be part of the general population; scientific population studies of supplements don't apply to you! You're an athlete and an exception to the rules.**

Many recommendations for supplements may be logical from a theoretical basis or from small studies. Thus, many supplements are without a robust scientific basis.

According to Professor Marina Heinon of the University of

Helsinki, 90% of health claims made by dietary supplements are incorrect [2].

FDA Regulations

In the U.S., the Food and Drug Administration (FDA) overseas the safety of food, drugs, and cosmetics. The rules they have promulgated regarding drugs that are intended to treat disease are far different than the rules regarding dietary food supplements. Today, the FDA usually requires a new drug to show superiority to the current standard of care using human prospective randomized studies. For a new drug to show 10% superiority usually requires a minimum of 400 patients.

According to *Forbes* magazine, the average cost of developing a new drug is at least $4 billion [3].

The costs of developing and bringing food supplements to market are minimal. No government approval is needed to make and sell a dietary food supplement, so caveat emptor—buyer beware. Canadian investigators using DNA barcoding tested 44 bottles of popular supplements sold by 12 companies. They found that 33% were not what they claimed to be [4].

Levels of Scientific Evidence

Level I—Prospective randomized trials agree—the most reliable information.

Level II—At least one prospective randomized trial is positive, but possibly imperfect design; disagreement in controlled studies—reliable information.

Level III—Case studies, retrospective data, historical data; possibly helpful information.

Level IV—Case studies, limited numbers, controversial information.

Level V—Expert opinion, controversial information, bodybuilding tradition, scientific theory.

In my medical practice, I'm required to use Level I or II evidence-based treatments for my sick patients. If this information is not available, then I use Level III or IV information; however, insurance companies frequently won't cover therapy based on Level III or IV data. What is written on a medication's package insert, and what insurance companies will pay for, is always Level I or II evidence. Many supplements lack data because data is too expensive to obtain, and the studies are done with small numbers of subjects over a short period of time.

Listed below are mostly over-the-counter supplements that you can purchase at vitamin shops and grocery stores. There are a few prescription drugs also included in this list as well.

Whey Protein (Level I)—Yes

Whey protein and casein are the proteins found in cow's milk. When renin is added to milk, the casein and whey separate, leaving the whey protein in solution and the casein solidifying into cheese. Both products are used in making protein supplements.

Whey protein is rapidly absorbed. Whey protein supplementation before and after resistance training sessions provide significantly greater improvement in exercise recovery both 24 and 48 hours post-exercise than found in subjects ingesting a placebo [5].

There are multiple studies showing that whey protein rapidly stimulates protein synthesis and increases muscle hypertrophy. Whey protein is best taken early post-exercise [6]. This is not controversial—**whey protein after exercise will help you build and maintain muscle.**

According to the EFSA Panel on Dietetic Products, Nutrition and Allergies [7], a cause-and-effect relationship has not been established between the consumption of whey protein and growth or maintenance of muscle mass over and above the well-established role of protein on the claimed effect. This complex language simply states that any source of protein will do. However, there's more to protein supplements and foods than just amino acids. You need to be careful which protein powder you choose; some of the popular protein products may contain relatively high amounts of cadmium, arsenic, lead, and mercury, and these are not listed on the package [8].

I recommend whey powders from grass-fed, antibiotic-free cows. Cows that are fed high-grain diets have a higher incidence of metabolic disorders related to the buildup of several toxic and inflammatory compounds, as well as changes in amino acid profiles in their digestive fluids, as compared to cows on low-grain diets. Having these metabolic complications (and the subsequent need for antibiotics) negatively affects the quality of dairy products produced, including the whey protein found in milk [9].

Why do farmers in the U.S. feed their cows grain? Farmers have turned to grains, such as corn, due to convenience and money. They confine cows to feedlots, feed them grains and also antibiotics and the enzymes necessary to digest grains since cows are normally unable to digest grains! The cows rapidly gain weight and yield a higher return on investment (more money). The quality of the milk may suffer.

Fish Oil (Level II)—Yes

Fish oil contains two essential omega-3 fatty acids that our bodies need and must obtain from food: docosahexaenoic acid (DHA), and eicosapentaenoic acid (EPA). These essential fatty acids are present in salmon, mackerel, sardines, flaxseeds, chia seeds, and walnuts. You need them.

Populations with high intakes of omega-3 (n3) polyunsaturated fatty acids (such as the Inuit) have low rates of heart disease. This observation has increased the interest in the possible benefit of fish oils [10]. Fish oil concentrate administered at high doses can reduce levels of triglycerides in patients with HIV and hypertriglyceridemia [11].

Other types of omega-3 supplements, such as flax seeds, appear to improve lipid blood levels [12] and are beneficial.

Negative fish oil data comes from a study that evaluated prostate cancer prevention in men taking selenium and vitamin E [13]. The study was negative but did reveal an increased prostate cancer risk in men with higher blood levels of long chain polyunsaturated fatty acids. This was based on a single blood test and was neither randomized nor prospective (Level III or IV).

Furthermore, taking fish oil supplements did not improve the natural history of patients with known coronary risk factors [14].

There are multiple studies that *do* show that a combination of fish oil and exercise increases protein synthesis in muscle cells and improves insulin sensitivity [15, 16].

Fish oil has anabolic properties and is useful in building muscle despite not being able to improve heart disease and possibly increasing prostate cancer risk. The choice is yours. I take fish oil.

Creatine (Level II)—Yes

Creatine makes more ATP in the mitochondria available for muscular activity, and this longer duration of muscle contraction enhances the power of athletes over a short period of time [17].

Creatine is not important for endurance athletes.

Taking approximately 20 grams of creatine per day over a seven-day period shows a measurable increase in power production during short-duration resistance exercises to muscle failure.

Creatine has not been shown to improve long-duration endurance exercise. Elevated muscle creatine enhances exercise performance by matching ATP supply to ATP demand.

An increase in body weight from one to two pounds is common after one week of creatine supplementation due to an increase in intracellular water.

There is little data on long-term creatine use. Creatine allows users to train more intensely. Few adverse side effects have been found with creatine use in healthy individuals [18].

Furthermore, a recent prospective study performed at the University of Regina, Saskatchewan, Canada in 2015 [19] showed that the addition of creatine supplementation realized improvements in both bone mineral density and muscle growth in older adults doing resistance training.

If you have a history of renal dysfunction, you should not take creatine, as it will increase the serum creatinine that your physician uses to measure your renal function.

I recommend a maintenance dose of 5 grams per day, along with frequent vacations from use, for older adults.

DHEA (Level III)—Still a Question; Possibly Yes

Dehydroepiandrosterone (DHEA) is a commercially available supplement aimed at improving libido and well-being. There is little evidence to support the use of DHEA for this purpose. DHEA is a precursor element for the production of androgens and estrogens in non-reproductive tissues.

Levels of DHEA decline with age. It has been postulated that restoring the circulating levels of DHEA to those that are found in young people may have anti-aging effects and improve well-being and sexual function. There is no randomized prospective scientific data to support this.

There is some positive data in patients with adrenal insufficiency. Studies of DHEA therapy in patients with adrenal insufficiency suggest that this group is the most likely to derive health benefits from DHEA supplementation.

There is one interesting positive study [20] by Yen, et al. In this study, men and women over the age of fifty took 50 mg of DHEA daily. DHEA levels rose to those of young adults within two weeks.

The subjects then had their immune systems assessed through the measurement of lymphocytes, T cells, and natural killer cells. The DHEA increased the levels of these cells by 67% in men and 84% in women.

A follow-up study using 100 mg of DHEA showed that the subjects also experienced gains in lean body mass as well as an increase in muscular strength. Male subjects also experienced a significant decrease in body fat. There is also evidence of benefit for women with post-menopausal bone density loss and with depressed patients [21, 22].

There are no long-term studies of elderly subjects taking 100 mg of DHEA daily. I take this supplement; caveat emptor.

Testosterone (Level I)—Yes, But Only With An Expert; Controlled Substance

According to the U.S. Library of Medicine and the U.S. Institute of Health, testosterone is a hormone made by the testicles in men. It's the most important androgen (male) hormone in the body. Women produce a smaller amount, converting estrogen to testosterone by way of the enzyme aromatase. Testosterone is essential for both men and women. Androgens, such as testosterone, are often referred to as steroids or anabolic steroids.

Testosterone is important for:

- Keeping bones and muscles strong

- Making sperm

- Maintaining sex drive

- Making red blood cells

- Feeling well and having energy in general.

As you become older, testosterone levels slowly drop. This can lead to various symptoms, including:

- Low sex drive

- Problems having an erection

- Low sperm count

- Sleep problems, such as insomnia

- Decrease in muscle size, strength, and bone density

- Increase in body fat

- Depression

- Trouble concentrating

Who Should Try Testosterone Therapy?

To help assess whether testosterone therapy is right for you, your doctor will likely do the following:

- Measure your free and total testosterone levels one or more times as well as estradiol levels and other essential blood tests as described below.

- Make sure there are no other causes of your symptoms. These include side effects from medicines, thyroid problems, depression, or overuse of alcohol.

If your testosterone level is low, your doctor will discuss the risks and benefits of testosterone therapy and how this therapy may help you.

In my opinion, most physicians are *not* knowledgeable regarding testosterone and are hesitant to prescribe testosterone, which is a controlled substance. They will tell you that the signs and symptoms of low testosterone are part of the normal aging process.

If you wish to age *normally*, you're reading the wrong book. In men and women over 40 years of age, maintaining sufficient levels of testosterone in the blood is an important part of building muscle, increasing activity level, losing body fat, and increasing endurance. Your blood levels should be checked by an expert—total testosterone, free testosterone, estradiol, IGF1, TSH, lipid profile with LDL subsets, PSA, CBC, and CMP.

If your testosterone levels are low, the best replacement is by way of a testosterone injection since this is similar to the testosterone made by your body. It does not require liver activation, as do testosterone pills and creams, and does not add stress to your liver.

Testosterone and estradiol levels must be monitored frequently because some of the added testosterone will be aromatized to estrogen.

Testosterone is a hormone and a ligand (a molecule that binds to another, usually larger, molecule). Like any other ligand, in chronic excess, cells may become immune to its actions and cause pathology. There are no scientific data linking testosterone to either prostate or breast cancer. However, testosterone accelerates the growth of prostate cancer, should it already be present. Testosterone has benefits for older adult men [23]. Among a group of men in the Veterans Administration healthcare system who underwent coronary angiography and had a low serum testosterone level, the use of testosterone therapy was associated with an increased risk of adverse outcomes [24]. This VA study demonstrated a 5.8% increased risk of cardiovascular events over a period of three years. Despite the improvement in sexual function, bone mineral density, decreased body fat, increased strength, improved lipid profiles, and decreased insulin resistance, there is an increased incidence of mortality with testosterone supplementation. This poorly controlled study did not evaluate the type of testosterone supplements, estradiol levels, nor free and total testosterone blood levels. **No blood tests were required after the initial finding of a low total testosterone.** This 5.8% increase in this study of men can likely be attributed to elevated estradiol levels, a known cardiac risk factor.

An 83,000-patient study of European veterans showed that normalization of testosterone levels with testosterone supplements only showed cardiovascular benefits [25]. The cardiac benefits of testosterone have been shown in more than one scientific study [26].

Testosterone by injection remains controversial because there are no prospective randomized studies—level 1 or 2 data. These important studies will never be done by the pharmaceutical companies because a natural hormone made by your body cannot be patented, so there is no financial incentive to do the study. Drug companies will not study a drug they cannot patent and profit from.

Human Chorionic Gonadotropin (hCG) (Level IV)—No for Weight Loss, No for Fat Loss

The peptide hCG is indicated in men to prevent testicular atrophy associated with the long-term use of testosterone. Under normal conditions, the testicles produce testosterone. If testosterone levels drop and are supplemented with exogenous testosterone in order to maintain normal blood levels, the brain detects the change and stops stimulating the testicles (by way of luteinizing hormone, LH) to produce testosterone.

In this setting, the testicles may atrophy from disuse. The addition of hCG stimulates the testicles to continue producing testosterone (hCG mimics LH) and thus prevents atrophy. In males, hCG alone, without testosterone supplementation, can increase the production of testosterone by the testicles. Thus, hCG can be used alone to restore normal levels. In many states, hCG is not a controlled substance. However, the need for medical experts is essential if you wish to increase testosterone.

The use of hCG in women is not essential since women do not have testicles and hCG will not increase testosterone production. There is no evidence in non-pregnant women that hCG will increase the use of fat as a source for cellular energy. In both women and men, the controversy is really regarding weight loss and the hCG diet.

Since the hCG diet contains 500 to 1,000 calories per day, all the benefits achieved on the hCG diet can be attributed to caloric restriction. A review study refuting the hCG diet has been published in the *American Journal of Clinical Nutrition*, concluding that hCG is neither safe nor effective as a weight loss aid [27]. There is no evidence that hCG will selectively increase fat loss or preserve muscle mass during weight reduction.

Beta-Hydroxy Beta-Methylbutyrate (HMB) (Level III)—Yes

HMB (Bhydroxyl Bmethylbutyrate) is an effective supplement for adults to increase lean body mass according to a meta-analysis and multiple scientific studies [28]. HMB and a mixture of other branched-chain amino acids improve protein metabolism and increase lean body mass in elderly and chronically ill subjects.

HMB benefits people who exercise vigorously (defined as three weeks or more of resistance training two or more times a week) [29].

HMB has data supporting its use to augment lean mass and strength gains with resistance training. The benefits of this supplement have been confirmed by meta-analysis.

Vitamin D3 (Level II)—Yes

Vitamin D3 deficiency is common in the USA—41%, and can be as high as 82% in certain high-risk populations [30]. Vitamin D is essential to maintain your bone health, and it does much more than this. Vitamin D deficiency is associated with a higher risk of certain diseases—colon cancer [31], cardiovascular disease [32], and autoimmune diseases [33]. According to the National Institute of Health office of dietary supplements, older adults are at an increased risk of developing vitamin D insufficiency. Older skin cannot synthesize vitamin D efficiently. Many adults spend little time outdoors, and they may have inadequate dietary intake of this vitamin. Your body is designed to manufacture vitamin D when sunlight shines on your skin. In the presence of a low vitamin D level, your body may lose bone density, and you will be at a risk for bone fractures. The loss of height in many older adults is due to the loss of bone density and the decrease in size of the bones in the spine. Exercise is also important in maintaining bone density in the weight-bearing bones of your body. Many adults in the United States with hip fractures have low serum vitamin D levels <30 nmol/L (<12 ng/mL). Osteoporosis is a pathological loss of bone density (2.5 standard deviations from a healthy bone, as measured on a DEXA scan) requiring medical treatments to prevent fracture. Osteopenia is a much more common condition—less bone loss then osteoporosis—and can be treated with non-prescription calcium and vitamin D supplements and weight-bearing exercise. Weight-bearing exercise includes walking, running, lifting, and dancing. Swimming will not strengthen your bones.

Medium Chain Triglycerides (MCT) (Level III)—Yes for Body Fat Loss

Medium chain triglycerides (MCT) are made from coconut and palm kernel oils. They differ from the saturated fats found in meat and dairy owing to their ability to rapidly enter the blood circulation and go directly to the liver.

Normal fats must be digested slowly, requiring chylomicrons (lipoprotein particles that transport dietary lipids from the intestines to other locations in the body) and slow lymphatic transport. MCT are rapidly metabolized into an energy source, and less fat from this source is stored in fat cells—so less fat accumulates [34].

MCT cause significant weight loss, lower fat deposition, and decrease appetite due to increased satiety. More research needs to be done regarding the long-term benefits of MCT.

Branched-Chain Amino Acids—Yes if You Exercise and Add Whey Protein

The branched-chain amino acids are valine, leucine, and isoleucine. Many have believed that the oral intake of these 3 BCAAs during exercise will prevent muscle breakdown during exercise and produce a post-workout muscle building response. BCAAs do enhance muscle growth but only slightly better than control groups without BCAAs. There is no significant statistical benefit to taking BCAAs alone [35]. This is not the complete story. The reason BCAAs do not work is that they lack other essential amino acids. When the studies are repeated, adding 20 grams of whey protein to the BCAAs, the anabolic response doubled [36]. To ensure muscle building benefit immediately after resistance training, the athlete should take BCAAs and whey protein together.

Resveratrol (Level V)—Too Early to be Certain; Caveat Emptor

Resveratrol has become famous as the ingredient in red wine that will make you live longer [37]. Many experts claim that resveratrol will also prevent the metabolic diseases of aging and prevent cancer by gene activation.

Many studies have shown that resveratrol has anti-aging, anti-carcinogenic, and anti-inflammatory effects in laboratory animals. This might be relevant to humans, but human data is not yet available. The limited human clinical trials to date only attest to resveratrol's safety and bio-availability [38]. Resveratrol decreases luteinizing hormone (LH) and is used to treat Polycystic Ovarian Syndrome. Reducing LH in men could interfere with testicular function.

Soy (Level III)—Useful Protein Source for Some, Not All

Soy is a useful source of protein for some, but not all, and much research continues [39].

Soy products are frequently found in grocery stores throughout the U.S. and are mostly consumed by infants, vegetarians, and Asians. In Korea, Japan, China, and Indonesia, soy proteins are more popular. Soy protein, unlike other vegetable proteins, contains all the essential amino acids and is an important food.

Soy contains isoflavones, which are plant estrogens, and these have numerous effects on the human body that are not found in animal protein sources. Soy isoflavones are controversial and are currently being researched, since estrogens can alter cell function, including cell cycle, fertility, and ovarian function in animal studies.

In humans, soy products are commonly found in baby foods, and no negative effects have yet to be found in adults who were fed soy baby foods when they were young.

With regard to the cardiovascular benefits of soy proteins, there is a minor reduction in low-density lipoproteins (LDL).

The real potential danger of isoflavones occurs in breast tissue, where breast secretions and cell proliferation are increased—a potential sign of an increased risk of breast cancer.

In summary, soy products are good sources of protein and good sources of fiber for most people.

Statins and Red Rice Yeast (Level I)— These Prevent Heart Attacks in Patients With Coronary Artery Disease

Red rice yeast is an ancient Chinese and Japanese food and traditional medicine. It is obtained by cultivating fermented rice with a mold called monascus purpureus. This traditional remedy was used to invigorate the body.

In a 2006 Chinese prospective randomized study of 5,000 patients with coronary artery disease, a Chinese standardized red rice yeast product reduced the incidence of repeat heart attacks by 45% and reduced cardiac deaths by 31% [40].

The drug lovastatin (Mevacor), approved by the U.S. FDA to lower cholesterol and prevent heart attacks in patients with coronary artery disease, contains the identical compounds—monacolins—that are present in red rice yeast.

The 2014 guidelines of the American College of Cardiology recommended statins for anyone with existing coronary artery disease, an LDL of 190 mg/dl or higher, type 2 diabetes in those aged 40 to 70 years, and anyone in the 40 to 70-year-old group with a 7.5% risk of developing coronary artery disease. This last group of 7.5% risk is controversial and is Level IV evidence. I am over 70 years, and my LDL is slightly over 190 mg/dl, and I do not take a statin. However, I exercise and I have a healthy diet. I consider myself an athlete and not an average unhealthy American. In addition, using total LDL as a marker of cardiovascular health is flawed because it is only the small particle LDL that is harmful. LDL is discussed in other sections of this book regarding vegetarian diets and lipoproteins.

Coenzyme Q10 (CoQ10) (Level V)—Yes

Coenzyme Q10 is present in the mitochondria of every living cell in your body. The greater the metabolic activity of the cell, the greater the concentration of CoQ10.

According to the Mayo Clinic (mayoclinic.org), deficiencies of CoQ10 may cause heart failure and high blood pressure. There is good scientific evidence that treating these deficiencies with CoQ10 supplements is effective in improving chronic congestive heart failure and hypertension [41].

CoQ10 is a dietary supplement and is thus not under federal regulation, and since it's available over the counter, it's unlikely that any prospective randomized studies will be done. In general, randomized studies are expensive to do and are done only when a drug can be patented and thus enable pharmaceutical companies to have a return on their investment.

It's interesting to note that CoQ10 levels decrease with the use of cholesterol-lowering drugs (statins). Supplemental CoQ10 should be taken by everyone on statins. This is a good reason to use statins or any cholesterol-lowering supplements *only* where Level I and Level II data exist, as in the case of men with proven coronary artery disease and/or diabetes.

Coffee (Level III)—Yes

Despite what critics say, caffeine can be healthy. Early studies showing coffee as harmful were done when the harmful effects of smoking were not taken into consideration; most coffee drinkers at that time also smoked cigarettes.

According to the Mayo Clinic, coffee may protect you from

Parkinson's disease, diabetes, and liver cancer. Coffee improves cognitive function and memory and decreases the risk of depression by blocking the inhibitor neurotransmitter adenosine [42].

Caffeine is a fat burner and can increase adrenaline levels and release fatty acids from the fat tissues. Coffee can increase your metabolic rate by 3-11% [43]. A cup of coffee can improve your performance in the gym by 11-12% [44].

Probiotics (Level II)

Today there is much discussion of probiotics and little prospective randomized data. Probiotics are living, nonpathogenic bacteria or yeast ingested to benefit the gastrointestinal tract and/or vagina.

Probiotics are not regulated by the FDA or any other governmental agency and are available over the counter. Due to this liberal policy, there is little drug company interest in performing expensive randomized studies.

The most consistent data involves various strains of Lactobacillus [45]. *Lactobacillus rhamnosus GG* can reduce diarrhea. *LNCFM* can improve lactose intolerance. *L. casei Shirota* and *L. MM53* decrease gastroenteritis caused by rotavirus. *L. GR1* and *L. B54* can restore vaginal microflora and prevent urinary tract infections. Some strains help to maintain remission status in inflammatory bowel disease.

Randomized studies have been done with *S. boulardii* and *L. rhamnosus*, and labs showed improvement in diarrhea caused by antibiotics [46].

Over-the-Counter Fat Burners

The best thing about fat burner supplements is their name.

The "fat burner" concept is that there are substances which increase the use of fat as a source of energy for cells, causing one to lose body fat.

There are many supplements sold in stores called fat burners, for which there is little or no scientific information. These include Lcarnitine, DHEA, yohimbe, garcinia cambogia, and raspberry ketones.

Caffeine (Level I)—A True Fat Burner

In one controlled study, caffeine was found to have enhanced the endurance of long-distance bicyclists. This was due to the combined effects of caffeine on lipolysis (the breakdown of fats by hydrolysis to release fatty acids) and its positive influence on nerve impulse transmission.

In the bicyclists who had caffeine, there was a greater rate of lipid metabolism compared to the decaffeinated treatment group. Calculations of carbohydrate (CHO) metabolism from respiratory exchange data revealed that the subjects oxidized roughly 240 grams of CHO in both trials. Fat oxidation was significantly higher ($P < 0.05$) during the caffeine group than in the decaffeinated group. On average, the participants rated their effort (perceived exertion scale) during the caffeine trial to be significantly easier ($P < 0.05$) than the demands of the decaffeinated group [47].

Caffeine works by increasing the rate of fatty acid metabolism. If you drink coffee before you exercise, you'll use more calories from fat; thus, you will truly burn fat.

Ephedrine (Level II)—A Fat Burner

Ephedrine is a stimulant (sympathomimetic amine) that increases dopamine and noradrenaline in the brain [48]. Ephedrine promotes short-term weight loss [49]. Ephedrine is an FDA-controlled substance and is limited to the treatment of diseases such as asthma, bronchitis, and allergies.

Caffeine and ephedrine are synergistic in weight loss effect [50]. Ephedrine, caffeine, and aspirin taken together are a popular combination used by bodybuilders to cut down on body fat before a competition.

Green Tea Extract (Level II)—Fat Burner

Green tea promotes fat oxidation beyond that attributable to its caffeine content. Green tea extract contains catechins (a type of disease-fighting flavonoid and antioxidant) that play a role in the control of body composition via sympathetic activation of thermogenesis, fat oxidation, or both [51].

Irisin (Level IV)—Fat Burner

Irisin is a hormone produced naturally by muscle tissue and exercise that converts white storage fat to energy-producing brown fat [52]. More data is needed. It is available as an oral supplement.

CHAPTER 17
Estrogen Replacement— Essential for Most Perimenopausal and Postmenopausal Women—the Debacle of 2004—Yes, in the Absence of Breast Cancer—Level II Data

The use of estrogen supplements at menopause is extremely important and has been completely misrepresented in the public media. On July 9, 2002, the first Women's Health Initiative (WHI) study reported an increased risk of breast cancer and cardiovascular events in women on hormone replacement with Pempro—a mixture of synthetic estrogen (Premarin) and synthetic progesterone (Provera) [1]. Millions of women worldwide had been taking Prempro, and this information was turned into a campaign against hormone replacement therapy [2]. In 2004, a second WHI WHO report found that Premarin (estrogen) alone decreased the risk of breast cancer and did not increase the risk of cardiovascular complications [3]. It was the synthetic progestin Provera that was dangerous. This information has been ignored, and to this day many believe estrogen replacement therapy in any form is harmful. It is now proven that early estrogen replacement will decrease coronary atherosclerosis [4].

The benefits of estrogen replacement include relief of hot flashes, increased bone density in refractory bone loss, increased health and longevity [5]. Post-menopausal women (low estrogen) do not obtain the benefits of exercise as well as men [6]. In the absence of a high familial risk for breast cancer, estrogen replacement for perimenopausal and postmenopausal women is essential.

Katherine's Story

Katherine is a 55-year-old married female. She had a full-time job with a marketing company and worked five days a week. She had multiple new symptom complaints—bone pains in her back and hips, headaches, fuzzy thinking, muscle pains, insomnia, and hot flashes. She had stopped having menstrual periods one year ago. In view of these new symptoms, I was compelled to evaluate her with blood tests and a bone density scan.

All of Katherine's routine tests were normal except for an elevated total cholesterol of 250 mg/dl and a low estradiol level of 10 pg/ml. Her DEXA scan revealed osteopenia. Her primary physician had placed her on Crestor—a statin to reduce cholesterol levels— despite the fact that she had no family history of heart disease, nor any personal history of diabetes, chest pain, or heart disease. She had no family history of cancer, and her last mammogram was normal. She was not diabetic. Her lipid profile in my office was otherwise normal. I ordered a coronary artery CT scan of her heart to check for calcium-containing plaques in her coronary arteries, and essentially no calcium plaques were found.

I immediately discontinued her Crestor and placed her on a bioidentical estrogen and progesterone. Within four weeks, all her symptoms disappeared.

CHAPTER 18
Women are Complicated—
Hormone Replacement Therapy

Women are complex because their hormones are constantly changing.

Normal 28-Day Menstrual Cycle

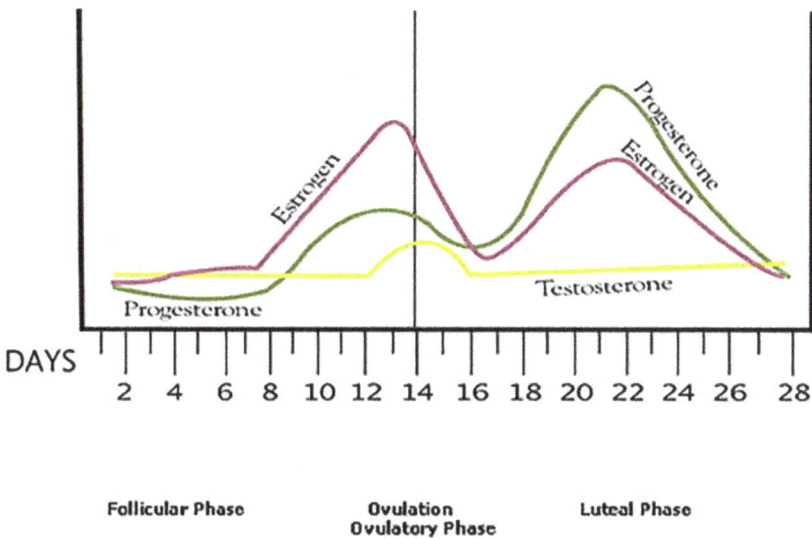

DAYS

2 4 6 8 10 12 14 16 18 20 22 24 26 28

Follicular Phase   Ovulation   Luteal Phase
                      Ovulatory Phase

In addition to the menstrual changes, there are age related changes. By age 50, women lose 30% of their estrogen and 75% of their progesterone. These changes in hormone levels cause women to experience a multitude of physical and emotional changes that men do not experience. With the addition of pregnancy, the list increases. We will attempt to explain the many complex changes women experience by focusing on estrogen and progesterone.

During day 1, the menstrual flow is greatest, and the estrogen blood level is low. The estrogen level gradually increases to its highest level on the day of ovulation—usually day 14. The estrogen level starts to decrease but reaches a second slightly lower peak on day 21. The drop continues to day 1 and starts all over if there is no conception [1]. There is a strong correlation between estrogen and mood in young women [2].

The physical shape of a woman's body is determined by the amount of estrogen she produces. Estrogen abundance causes more breast development and shorter stature due to earlier bone closure.

Estrogen and Balance Theory

The female body produces 4 types of estrogen: E1-Estrone, E2-Estradiol, E3-Estriol and E4-Estetrol. E2 is the predominant estrogen during reproductive years by serum levels and activity. Estrone is dominant during menopause. Estriol is dominant during pregnancy. Estetrol is made only during pregnancy. These 4 estrogens are synthesized from androgens by the enzyme aromatase. There are other minor estrogens as well. E1 and E2 are produced every day. Progesterone is produced only during the two weeks after ovulation. In the absence of ovulation, there is no progesterone produced, and estrogen remains unopposed or "dominant". The

196

symptoms and signs of estrogen dominance: breast discomfort, uterine wall thickening, headache, anxiety, depression, fluid retention, and food cravings. This concept of balance is a theory. The symptoms of estrogen dominance can be considered a medical syndrome. Unopposed estrogen does not cause breast cancer as clearly shown in the Women's Health Initiative.

The Benefit of Estrogen Replacement: Heart—Breast—Brain

Heart

Estrogen protects the heart as does bioidentical progesterone. Estrogen replacement therapy in women 50 to 74 years of age decreases their risk of a myocardial infarction—commonly known as a heart attack [3]. Heart disease is the leading cause of death worldwide, and it accelerates in postmenopausal women [4]. Estrogen has a protective effect on the cardiovascular system [5]. The non-bioidentical progestin Provera causes coronary artery spasm that increases cardiovascular complications while bioidentical progesterone does not [6].

Breast

In regard to breast cancer risk, the data is not so clear. Epidemiologic studies do not control all the variables. What is known from randomized clinical data is that non-bioidentical estrogen (Premarin) plus the artificial progestin (Provera) is associated with increases in breast cancer while the same estrogen alone in postmenopausal women is associated with a reduced risk of breast cancer [7]. The value of progesterone use with estrogen replacement is that progesterone reduces the risk of endometrial cancer by preventing the endometrial cell proliferation caused by estrogen. The data regarding breast cancer risk and bioidentical progesterone has been reviewed, and no increased risk has been found over a 5-year period [8].

Brain

Estrogen has neuroprotective and anti-aging properties. Despite lifestyle related stresses, aging is the most important risk factor for dementia [World Health Statistics 2017]. In addition, women live longer than men [9]. Age-related neurodegenerative diseases are different in men and women. Parkinson's Disease occurs more frequently in men. Alzheimer's Disease occurs more frequently in post-menopausal women than in men. In an age matched memory study, women are better than men [10]. This data suggests that the time of estrogen exposure may be an important variable. In animal models, decreasing estrogen enhances neurodegenerative disease. The Women's Health Initiative showed that estrogen replacement helps the healthy brain—there was a limited time period around menopause that estrogen was beneficial. Progesterone is also important for normal brain function since progesterone receptors are present in all neurologic brain cells [10]. Progesterone is therapeutic in the animal model of Parkinson's disease and traumatic brain injury. It reduces inflammatory markers and promotes myelin formation. Estrogen receptors and progesterone receptors are present throughout the brain. This is how they regulate higher cognitive functions such as mood, emotions, and motor skills [11]. During aging, there is a decline in neuronal function, a decline in sex hormone levels, and an increase in neurodegenerative diseases. Estrogen is neuroprotective.

Bioidentical Progesterone Capsules

Bioidentical progesterone capsules are available today and are useful in hormone replacement. The main reason for women on estrogen replacement to take bioidentical progesterone is that estrogen alone will lead to symptoms of estrogen dominance. It is also essential to prevent endometrial hyperplasia. Blood levels will accurately measure the results. Unlike birth control pills and non-bioidentical products, bioidentical progesterone does not increase the risk of a blood clot. Before starting estrogen and/or progesterone replacement therapy, you should see your doctor for a complete medical evaluation. Follow the medical guidelines for pelvic exams and mammograms. It is reasonable to have a pelvic ultrasound to measure the thickness of your uterus since any estrogen-like product will cause uterine thickening. Your doctor may require blood tests, and these should include measurements of your estrogen (E2), progesterone, sex hormone binding globulin (SHBG), testosterone, complete blood count (CBC), and complete metabolic profile (CMP).

Young Women—No Periods—Amenorrhea

There are 2 possible causes. In primary amenorrhea, there is no ovulation because the body is not producing enough estrogen and progesterone. Blood tests will confirm this as well as low follicle stimulating hormone (FSH) and low SHBG. The treatment is hormone replacement with bioidentical estrogen and progesterone. In secondary amenorrhea, there is no ovulation and little progesterone-estrogen, and SHBG is normal. The treatment is progesterone.

Bioidentical progesterone is best given by capsules. The precise dose varies according to the amount of estrogen dominance. Most women will need 50 mg at lunchtime and 100 mg at bedtime. The optimal dose of progesterone occurs when there are no symptoms of estrogen dominance: no water retention, no breast tenderness, and no insomnia. This is a clinical determination.

Ideal Blood Work After Hormone Replacement

In regard to ideal blood work—6 to 8 hours after hormone replacement: estradiol (E2) 50-250pg/ml; progesterone over 5 ng/ml; and SHBG under 90nmol/L.

Young Women With Abnormal Uterine Bleeding

The first test is a pregnancy test to rule out pregnancy. In ovulating women with insufficient progesterone, there are two different patterns of bleeding: normal flow but earlier—day 18 to 24; spotting day 21 to 26. The earlier the bleeding, the earlier the decrease in progesterone. The cause of the lower progesterone level is a problem in the cells (corpus luteum) of the unfertilized egg. The treatment is progesterone replacement.

Premenstrual Syndrome—PMS

Premenstrual syndrome is a group of symptoms that occur in women between ovulation and menstrual bleeding. The symptoms include mood changes, tender breasts, food cravings, fatigue, irritability and depression. PMS is associated with a decrease in progesterone in the blood and an associated decrease in the brain of the neurotransmitter GABA [12]. PMS is best treated with progesterone one day before the symptoms start, or approximately on day 15, and continue until menstruation.

CHAPTER 19
The Medical Management of Obesity— The Doctor's Point of View— Level II Data

The National Health and Nutrition Survey results (NHANES, 1999) estimate that 61% of U.S. adults are either overweight or obese. Adult obesity nearly doubled during the 14 years of the study, increasing to 27% [1].

Obesity is an independent risk factor for early mortality. Overall mortality begins to increase with BMI levels greater than 25 and increases most dramatically as BMI levels surpass 30 [2]. The longer the duration of obesity, the higher the risk [3].

Obesity predisposes a person to coronary artery disease by increasing your blood pressure (hypertension), producing abnormal lipids, and increasing insulin resistance. In addition to heart disease, obesity causes sleep apnea and degenerative joint disease.

A modest weight loss of 10% of your body weight will reduce insulin resistance, lower blood pressure, and decrease abnormal lipid production [4].

This book recommends diet and exercise together as the best treatment for obesity. In addition to diet and exercise, other treatments can include pharmacotherapy, supplements, hormone replacement therapy, behavior therapy, and surgery. The surgical approach is discussed in another section.

A low-calorie diet of 500 calories below your maintenance calorie level will reduce total body weight by 8% over three to twelve months. A very low-calorie diet totaling 800 calories per day will produce a very rapid loss of weight. This extremely low-calorie diet cannot be maintained in the long term and after one year is not superior to the maintenance-minus-500-calorie-diet approach [6].

Exercise at 60% to 85% of estimated maximum heart rate over three to seven 30 to 60-minute sessions per week produces a modest amount of weight loss of three to six pounds in one year [7].

The benefits of exercise cannot be measured in weight loss alone, as discussed in other sections of this book. The benefit of diet and exercise together provides greater weight loss than either one alone, as shown by studies of up to two years' duration [8].

Behavior therapy consists of behavior modification directed toward diet and exercise. This means counseling the patient regarding a healthy lifestyle, setting goals, self-monitoring toward these goals, and willpower. It's difficult to evaluate behavior therapy alone, since the goal is to get the patient on a diet and exercising.

The final subject is drug therapy. The role of drug therapy in obesity is controversial since most patients regain their lost weight once the drug is discontinued. The decision to initiate drug therapy requires careful evaluation of risks and benefits. Drugs can help a patient lose body fat when used with both diet and exercise. Candidates for drug therapy include those who are unable to diet and/or exercise; those with a BMI greater than 30 kg/m2; those with a BMI of 27 to 29.9 kg/m2, with comorbidities such as hypertension, diabetes, and coronary artery disease; those for whom gastrointestinal bypass surgery is being considered; and those in whom essential surgery cannot be performed, technically owing to the high risk caused by morbid obesity.

The Doctor's Dilemma—
The Story of Officer Tom

Tom is a 42-year-old police officer initially weighing 245 pounds and measuring six feet in height. His initial BMI of 33.2 placed him in the obese category. He had gained 50 pounds over the last three years, and his recent physical exam and blood tests revealed the onset of hypertension, hyperlipidemia and early type 2 diabetes. His chief had recently required that all officers pass a fitness test designed to simulate a foot pursuit and give aid to an injured officer. Tom did not pass the fitness test, and his job was in jeopardy. Tom's goal was to pass the test and lose 30 pounds. I placed him on a low-calorie diet of 1000–1200 calories per day—200 g protein and 50 g carbohydrate. The proteins were confined exclusively to beef, chicken, fish, lean pork, and eggs. The carbohydrates were restricted to berries, salads, and vegetables. Tom was instructed to take the appetite suppressant phentermine. He was monitored by weekly clinic visits, and Tom kept a daily diary of his diet and activity. After ten weeks, he had lost 30 pounds and his BMI had dropped to 29.2. He was no longer obese. His blood tests and blood pressure showed improvement, and he was able to pass the fitness test. Was this a good result? Would statins and pills for hypertension and diabetes be a better option? Tom was healthier and happy. The ultimate benefit depends upon what happens next. He had the essential requirements for success—a goal to lose 30 pounds, a daily diary to monitor success, the discipline to follow the program, and clinic visits where he was in the company of like-minded people. Can Tom continue this program in the future? Are long-term appetite suppressants his best option?

This is the doctor's dilemma of rapid success with a low-calorie diet and appetite suppressants. Many patients are unable or unwilling to exercise and maintain healthy diets. If Tom had measured his percentages of body fat and muscle mass, he would have found a loss of muscle mass that accompanied his 30-pound weight loss. The questions regarding the best treatment for Tom remains answered since he has achieved his goals and is content. We do not live in an ideal world, and human behavior, as discussed earlier, is governed by both emotions (fast thinking) and objectivity (slow thinking). The doctor cannot monitor your daily behavior nor take you to the grocery store nor take you to the gym. My guess is that Tom may choose to remain on phentermine for a long period of time.

The Appetite Suppressants

Phentermine—Phendimetrizine

There are seven main FDA-approved drug options used in obesity treatment. For a new drug to be approved by the FDA, it must be tested against a placebo and show weight loss greater or equal to 5% weight loss at one year, or show that 35% of patients achieve 5% weight loss, and must achieve twice the loss of the placebo patients. A commonly used drug is phentermine, owing to its efficacy and low price. This drug was approved by the FDA in 1959, and since generic, there has been little research done on this drug. Phentermine is an amphetamine-like drug that suppresses appetite by acting on several brain nuclei in the hypothalamus. Outside the brain, phentermine causes fat cells to break down fat by releasing epinephrine and norepinephrine. Phendimetrizine is very similar.

Diethylpropion

Diethylpropion is an amphetamine-like drug with minor sym-pathomimetic properties and with fewer stimulant effects than phentermine. The FDA approved diethylpropion in 1959 for treatment of obesity. A meta-analysis that assessed the use of diethylpropion for weight loss in obese individuals identified thirteen studies published between 1965 and 1983. Obese patients treated lost an average of 3 kg of additional weight compared with a placebo [9].

Diethylpropion's approval was based upon 69 patients randomized to diethylpropion 50 mg twice daily or placebo for six months. After this period, all participants received diethylpropion in an open-label extension for an additional six months. After the initial six months, the diethylpropion group lost an average of 9.8% of body weight versus 3.2% in the placebo group [10].

Common side effects of diethylpropion included insomnia, dry mouth, dizziness, headache, mild increases in blood pressure, palpitations, and rash.

Phentermine and Toperamide

The combination of phentermine and toperamide (Qsymia) is a powerful appetite suppressant and has been FDA-approved since 2012. Phentermine has been discussed and is FDA-approved for the short-term treatment of obesity, while topiramate is approved for non-weight-loss indications—seizure disorders and migraine therapy. The amount of weight loss achieved with combination therapy is of a greater magnitude than what could be achieved with either agent alone, and the combination may be taken for one year [11].

Lorcaserin

Lorcaserin (Belviq) is a 5-HT2c serotonin receptor agonist that decreases appetite by acting directly on these receptors in the brain. It cannot be used with any drug that alters the metabolism of serotonin, such as selective serotonin reuptake inhibitors, tricyclic antidepressants, bupropion, triptans, St. John's wort, tryptophan, drugs that impair metabolism of serotonin (including monoamine oxidase inhibitors), dextromethorphan, lithium, tramadol, antipsychotics, or other dopamine antagonists. Both lorcaserin and phentermine-topiramate have been approved for long-term weight loss based on one-year trials showing that, on top of recommendations to follow a calorie-restricted diet and to increase exercise, patients randomized to either drug lost more weight than patients randomized to placebo (3%), compared to lorcaserin (7%-8%) or phenteremine-toperamate (7%) [12]. These two drugs have been associated with side effects. Both drugs' labels include warnings about memory, attention, language problems, and depression. For lorcaserin, the label also warns of valvular heart disease and euphoria. And for phentermine-topiramate, the label warns of metabolic acidosis, increased heart rate, anxiety, insomnia, and elevated creatinine levels.

Orlistat

Orlistat is a lipase inhibitor that prevents fat absorption from the gut. It is available without a prescription. Orlistat prevents the absorption of 30% of ingested fat (Orlistat is dispensed as Xenical, 120-mg dose 3 times per day, daily. The side effects are substantial and include stool incontinence, fecal urgency, flatus, and fecal spotting. Orlistat is not the best treatment option owing to the unpleasant side effects.

Loraglitide

The fourth useful drug is loraglutide (Saxenda)—an injectable glucagon-like peptide that increases insulin production and decreases appetite. The side effects include nausea and diarrhea. It is useful in patients with both diabetes and obesity. This seems contradictory since one would expect that an increase in insulin would cause an increase in fat production. The mechanism of action is not completely understood but likely depends on direct uptake of loraglutide by the arcuate nucleus in the hypothalamus. The centrally projecting neurons in the arcuate nucleus are important in the regulation of appetite, and when activated, they inhibit feeding. These neurons are activated by leptin and insulin.

Naltraxone and Bupropion

The combination of Naltrexone and Bupropion is called Contrave. Naltrexone is an opioid antagonist that had been approved to treat opioid and alcohol dependency. It augments the action of Bupropion. Bupropion is a dopamine and norepinephrine reuptake inhibitor approved for depression and smoking addiction. It activates nuclei in the hypothalamus (brain) that decrease appetite and food cravings. This combination does not have any cardiac contraindications but does cause an increased rate of depression and suicide. One cannot drink alcohol or take opioid pain medications when taking Contrave.

Herbal treatments such as garcinia cambogia, have not been found useful in the treatment of obesity [14].

My criticism of my medical colleagues is simple. The FDA-approved use of every prescription drug for the treatment of obesity is preceded by the general statements, "when diet and exercise alone do not work" or "to be used with diet and exercise." This statement is never objectively controlled or quantified. How much exercise was performed? What was the calorie and macronutrient content of the diet? Was there a daily diary? Is the data a subjective, verbal report by the patient? My colleagues know that the benefits of prescription drug therapy occur only during drug therapy, and weaning patients off the drugs leads to weight gain in the absence of diet and exercise [15]. This is the benefit of short-term gain and the frustration of long-term weight regain. What is missing is that most weight loss physicians do not know how to transition a patient off weight loss medication and how to modify a diet as the patient's body changes. Many physicians do not know how to prescribe testosterone or estrogen when blood levels are low. No one wishes to change their comfortable lifestyle if they can achieve their goals by taking a pill. The successful treatment of obesity requires a long-term lifestyle change and a cultural change—knowledge, diet, supplements, and exercise. **There are only 4 things that increase metabolic rate and decrease appetite, and all four are essential tools for successful weight loss and permanent change in body composition—low-calorie diet with or without weight loss pill, exercise, increased protein and fat content of diet, median normal hormone levels.**

Successful Weight Loss Specifics

1. **Start a low-calorie diet higher in protein and fat and lower in carbohydrates, and include weight loss medication as needed to achieve body-fat loss.**

2. **As your body changes, wean off diet pills and increase exercise program.**

3. **Maintain median normal hormone levels and use supplements as needed—multivitamin, vitamin D3, and fish or krill oil.**

CHAPTER 20
In Theory, a Set Point Controls Your Body Weight

A body weight set point is a number—your weight—which your body maintains within a narrow range through a feedback and control system just like the thermostat in your home. The body weight set point involves your brain, gastrointestinal tract, circulating hormones/ligands/peptides, and fat cell mass. What is known is that in adults, body weight is maintained at a relatively stable level for long periods [1]. This observation is the basis for the set point theory. Information from the periphery is sent to a central controller located in the brain—hypothalamus. The controller uses this information to change or maintain food intake (hunger) and energy expenditure (metabolic rate) to correct any changes in body weight from this set point. This involves hormone/peptide signals from the hypothalamus, fat cell mass, and gastrointestinal tract.

The set point management of body weight is more effective in response to weight loss than to weight gain [1]. During weight loss, the body's metabolic rate—energy expenditure—decreases [2] and hunger increases.

After weight loss, changes in the circulating levels of several peripheral hormones, including the hunger hormone ghrelin, increase [4]. These hormone changes may remain in place for over one year [3]. This data helps to explain the results of the Minnesota starvation study [5], during which subjects decreased calorie intake by 68.9% and lost 66% of their initial fat mass after 24 weeks of dieting. After a period of refeeding with no restrictions, the subjects regained 145% of their original fat mass.

Leptin is another regulator of body weight or fat mass [6]. Leptin is made in fat cells and is proportional to the amount of fat present in the body. The hypothalamus uses this information to regulate the hunger hormone ghrelin and the metabolic rate to maintain the set point [1]. This is also the reason that diet alone will always fail, because diet alone will not change your weight set point, and the hormones/peptides stimulated by your brain will always win. This is a simple explanation. Diet pills such as Phentermine or Phendimetrizine work by counteracting the brain, increasing the metabolic rate and decreasing appetite.

Can you change your weight set point? There are no prospective controlled scientific studies that directly addresses this point. It is very difficult to completely control all the variables in humans. Most articles on set point change recommend a long, slow process of gradual weight loss. Medical weight loss programs with diet and prescription medication (diet pills) can counteract your brain's set point as long as you take the pills. Good examples of this are the drugs phendimetrazine and phentermine, which increase your metabolic rate because they are stimulants and decrease your hunger. This effectively counteracts your brain. This method, like diet alone, will fail when the pill is no longer taken, and the old set point remains.

Some expert obesity doctors believe it is not possible or practical to lower the set point without medical weight loss medication given continuously and indefinitely.

The Curious Case of Dr. M.R.

Dr. M.R. is a famous scientist known for his work in the field of obesity. He has meticulously studied the carbohydrate and insulin model of obesity. His problem is that he is obese and unable to lose body fat despite diet, moderate exercise, and his focused knowledge of nutrition. Dr. M.R. attributes his dilemma to his genetics since everyone in his family is obese, and he has given up in regard to changing his risk for chronic metabolic diseases. He has embraced his obesity and his current lifestyle and medications. This situation may be politically correct and the least stressful solution for many people. In my opinion, this is one of the reasons we wrote this book—to provide a wider range of information that many physicians do not have. The question, "Is obesity genetically determined?" has been asked by many scientists. The estimates of the inheritability of BMI vary from 47% to 80% [7].

Do obese mothers have obese babies? The answer is yes [8].

The most interesting studies come from obese women who, after bariatric surgery, deliver babies who weigh less than babies delivered by obese, comparable women who have not had bariatric surgery [9]. This data points to epigenetic environmental factors as the more important determinants of obesity. It is not so much the genes you were born with but the environmental factors that express certain genes and suppress others. I would guess that Dr. M.R. knew about this study since he had training in endocrinology and pediatrics.

In my opinion, you can lose weight and maintain the weight loss if you are able to change your lifestyle using all the tools and knowledge available—diet, exercise, supplements, and hormone replacement. Dr. M.R. was not interested in exercise and in his 6th decade had likely lost approximately 30% of his muscle mass and had a sedentary activity level. Like most 60-year-old men, he had a total testosterone level below the median level. I do not know his eating habits, but he had been obese his entire life.

My Answer

My answer is that exercise as well as increased fat and protein in a lower carbohydrate diet and supplements, including hormone replacement (HRT) if needed, are the missing ingredients. With exercise, higher fat/protein low-sugar diet, and HRT, the body fat set point will decrease because these lifestyle changes increase your metabolic rate and decrease your hunger—just like the weight loss pill. For pill-taking weight loss patients to maintain their lost weight, they must increase their exercise as they come off their weight loss pills and maintain a healthy diet and median, normal hormone levels. The other option is to take the weight loss pill indefinitely. This is another way of stating that your lifestyle must change, and diet, exercise, and supplements must become an important part of your new life that you continue indefinitely in order to maintain a lower body fat set point. If subjects are able to maintain weight loss for a period of one year, their bodies adapt and show increased levels of peptides that suppress appetite (GLP-1 and PYY3), while peptides that increase appetite decrease (ghrelin and GIP). This adaptation required one year and shows that the body set point can change [10].

CHAPTER 21
The Optimum Body Unification Theory: Autophagy and Anabolism

This is an attempt to explain how diet, exercise, supplements, and hormones work together to optimize your body. The longevity theories are helpful to tell us what is important in living a healthy life and to conceptualize the variables involved in optimal health. Much of this research has been conducted in animals and not in humans, and for that reason, this essay is theoretical. Statements without human studies will not be referenced, and human studies will be referenced.

There are two major processes that are going on in your body: anabolism, or the building up processes, and autophagy, the catabolic and "taking out the trash" processes. **They compete with each other and cannot occur at the same time, and both are necessary.**

Autophagy is the cellular process analogous to taking out the trash and finding reusable parts in the trash. Damaged cells are broken down, and the products are reused to build new cells. During times of nutrient deficiency—starvation—autophagy enables the body to survive by using an internal source for essential nutrients. An example of this is sleep. When you stop eating and go to sleep without a snack, your body enters a state of nutrient deficiency, or fasting, and the autophagic processes take over (*the mTOR kinases are suppressed*). Another example is the ketogenic diet when your body's fat cells are used to provide a source of energy for the other cells of the body and you lose body fat.

The competing processes to autophagy are the anabolic processes of cellular growth and cellular division involving protein synthesis and suppression of autophagy (*and the stimulation, or upregulation, of the mTOR kinases*). This occurs when you eat a lot of food and the body is in a nutrient-rich environment and when you do resistance exercises.

[The important variables at the cellular level are mTORC1, mTORC2, AMPK, and ULK1. MTORC1 is a kinase—it transfers a phosphate group from ATP to specific molecules that control cell growth and metabolism in response to nutrients and growth factors. MTORC1 regulates cell anabolic activity by upregulating/increasing protein synthesis. MTORC2 is a kinase that regulates the cytoskeleton inside cells. ULK1 is a kinase that activates autophagy—the process that removes damaged cells and regulates the degradation and recycling of cellular components. AMPK is an enzyme that regulates energy metabolism. AMPK mobilizes energy stores when energy is depleted and controls the expression of mTORC1, mTORC2 and ULK1.]

The mammalian target of rapamycin is called mTOR, and mTOR regulates cell growth, proliferation, and survival. MTOR is activated by food, glucose, lipids, amino acids, insulin, growth factors, and inflammatory cytokines [1]. MTOR is stimulated by muscle contraction-resistance exercise. Too much mTOR causes insulin resistance [2].

Optimum health requires a balance between the anabolic process and the catabolic (autophagy) process—both are necessary. In the mitochondrial theory of aging, it is the damaged mitochondria that decrease longevity. Autophagy is needed to remove damaged mitochondria and prolong longevity. *[In the presence of nutrient excess, mTOR stimulates cellular growth and inhibits autophagy. In nutrient-deficit, low-calorie diets, AMPK stimulates autophagy and suppresses mTOR1.]*

Increased mTOR occurs in human muscle in response to muscle contraction—an anabolic event [3]. Too much of either process causes metabolic disease. Too much mTOR leads to insulin resistance, increased fat production in the blood, and increased fat deposition in the liver. This causes obesity. Lipogenesis and insulin resistance lead to metabolic diseases such as type 2 diabetes. Too much autophagy leads to muscle loss, weakness, loss of bone density, and frailty.

We will now review how these two processes—autophagy and anabolism—are affected by our lifestyle: diet, exercise, supplements, and hormones.

Calorie restriction is the most effective way to increase lifespan in every animal model and in human studies. It involves reducing calorie intake by 20%-40% without malnutrition and causes a reduction of mTOR processes and insulin and an increase in the autophagic processes. Calorie excess increases mTOR, insulin, and subsequently cellular growth and all anabolic activity. Hormones and growth factors are also needed and regulate the speed of these activities.

Exercise

Resistance exercises in the presence of adequate nutrition increase the mTOR processes and stimulate skeletal muscle growth and increase strength. This continues with repeated exercise bouts as long as there is adequate recovery periods in between. Without appropriate recovery protein synthesis, anabolic growth does not occur. A recovery period of 2 or 3 days is suitable for gaining effects following exercise in the same muscle. Endurance training decreases mTOR processes (mediated by an increase in AMPK) and promotes autophagy.

You need both resistance exercise and cardiovascular exercise. The optimal sequence is resistance before cardiovascular exercise since mTOR is needed to build muscle and is suppressed by cardiovascular exercise

Diet

A high-protein diet increases mTOR and the anabolic processes. If you wish to build muscle or gain weight, you will need a high-protein and high-carbohydrate diet. Fasting, a lower calorie diet, and a low-carbohydrate ketogenic diet will lower mTOR and promote autophagy. Calorie reduction promotes longevity.

The Process of Autophagy

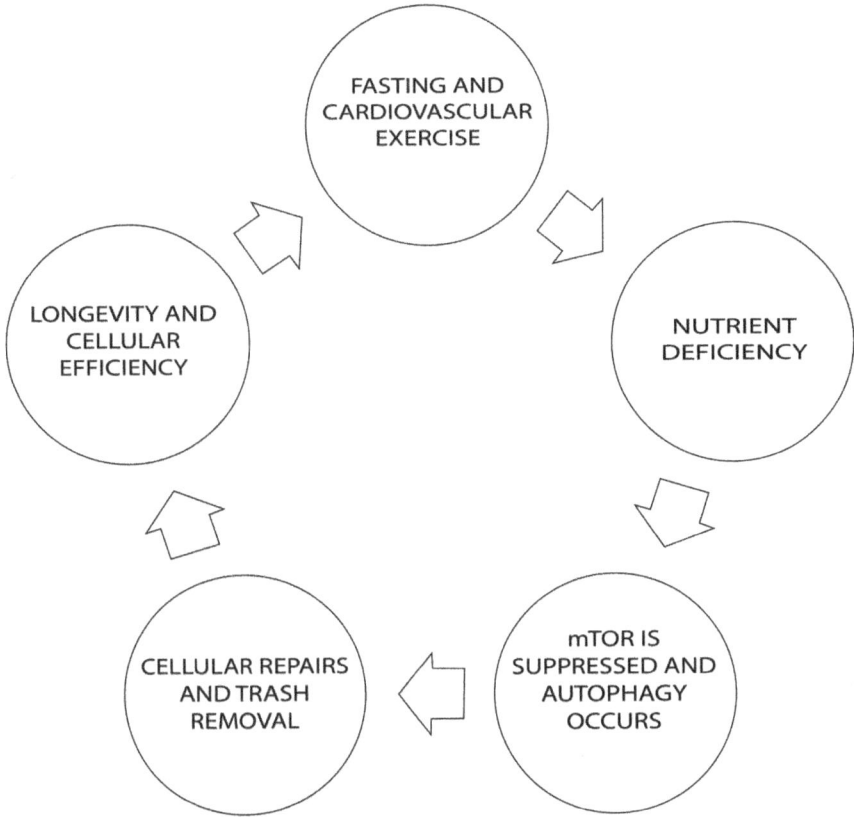

FASTING AND CARDIOVASCULAR EXERCISE

NUTRIENT DEFICIENCY

mTOR IS SUPPRESSED AND AUTOPHAGY OCCURS

CELLULAR REPAIRS AND TRASH REMOVAL

LONGEVITY AND CELLULAR EFFICIENCY

Anabolic Process

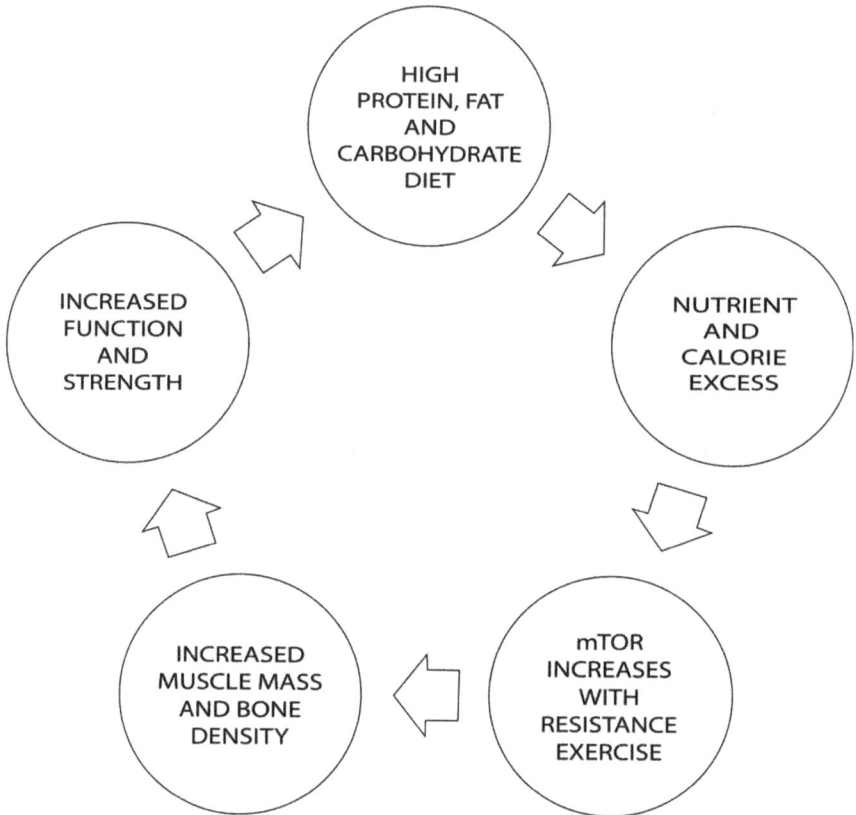

The best measure of balance between autophagy and anabolism is your body weight. If your weight is stable, you are in balance.

CHAPTER 22
Human Immunity—
Everything You Do

Everything you do will affect your immune function. Yes! Every single thing in your life matters. In this chapter, we will first define your immune system and then show how everything you do has an effect upon your ability to fight harmful microbes in the environment.

The human immune system protects us from harmful living things in the environment, too small to be seen, called microbes. Examples of microbes include bacteria and viruses. Where the environment enters our body, the immune system is very active. This includes our nose, mouth, lungs, sinuses and gastrointestinal tract. Microbes cover our body surfaces. The human immune response is complex and is designed to protect us from harmful microbes—pathogens. The immune system must be able to detect the harmful features of pathogens that are not part of our body (not host) and be able to destroy them safely. There are two genetic mechanisms for microbial recognition: the innate immune responses and the adaptive immune responses.

The innate immune system involves activating cells to create a general or nonspecific defense against common molecular patterns (viral or bacterial). The innate system is our rapid and our first line of defense and involves cells that eat or devour pathogens through phagocytosis. These cells include white blood cells such as monocytes, macrophage, and neutrophils. The adaptive immune system creates specific immune responses to pathogens (virus and bacterial structures). The adaptive response has memory cells that can activate quickly an immune response that had occurred in the past. The adaptive immune response involves T cells. The major anatomic components of the immune system include these sites: bone marrow, thymus gland, lymph nodes, spleen, and lymphatic ducts.

The Cells and Molecules of the Immune System

The cells in the immune system work together to identify, mark, and destroy pathogens. The **B cells** are lymphocytes that make a specific antibody against a specific pathogen—bacteria, virus, or malignant cell. Antibodies are proteins that target a specific marker on pathogens called antigens. **CD 8 killer T cells** (lymphocytes) directly contact and kill pathogens including cancer cells. **CD 4 helper T cells** (lymphocytes) help target CD 8 killer cells and help B cells as well. **Dendritic cells** digest pathogens and expose their surface proteins so other immune cells can recognize them. **Macrophage** engulf and destroy bacteria and other pathogens. There are also **Regulatory lymphocytes** that down regulate the cells of the immune system so that the inflammatory immune response does not harm the host. A continuous over reactive response can become an Autoimmune Disease. When immune cells work together, they communicate by releasing small proteins called **cytokines** that attach to cell surface receptors and modulate the activity of the immune cells and antibody production. The cytokines produce the "inflammation"—the clinical signs and symptoms of the immune response.

Nutrition and Immunity

The Immune System requires energy (calories) and specific nutrients: arginine, zinc, selenium, glutamine, and vitamins D, E and A [4].

The gastrointestinal tract associated lymphoid tissue (GALT) contains the largest number of immune system cells. When we eat, we ingest a large number of foreign antigens that require a near constant immune response and immune cell communication throughout the body. The human gastrointestinal tract is also home to over a trillion bacterial cells that interact with the immune system and are called the gut microbiome. The gut microbiome has nutritional requirements as well, and these are discussed in the chapter on Amazing Fiber. In summary, the GALT and the microbiome work together to keep our bodies healthy.

Obesity and the Immune System

Obesity impairs immune function, white blood cell counts, and cell mediated immune response [5]. T cell function is impaired [6]. Visceral fat—adipose tissue—is metabolically active and produces inflammatory molecules that alter the immune response [5]. Adipose tissue produces increased amounts of inflammatory molecules called adipokines: TNF—tumor necrosis factor, IL-6, and CRP—C-reactive protein. These inflammatory markers predispose to chronic metabolic diseases such as hypertension, type 2 diabetes, coronary artery disease, and dementia [4]. Leptin is another adipokine produced by fat cells that can inhibit natural killer T cells.

Exercise and the Immune System

Many epidemiologic studies show that regular physical activity enhances immune function and reduces the incidence of bacterial and viral infections, cancer, and chronic inflammation [7]. One or two hours of exercise may cause a transient decrease of lymphocytes in peripheral blood tests, but this is due to a redistribution of cells into the peripheral tissues and represents increased immune surveillance [7]. The proof of principle is that men ages 65 to 85 years who exercise regularly exhibited higher antibody responses to influenza vaccine compared to inactive control subjects [8]. Men who exercise regularly have greater T cell proliferation, higher natural killer cell cytotoxicity, and improved white blood cell phagocytosis [7]. Exercise has immunologic benefits at any age.

Aging and the Immune System

For most people, the immune system dramatically changes as we age and loses the ability to protect against infections and cancer [1]. Antibody responses to vaccines become impaired. T cells are impaired. There is loss of adaptive immunity and gain in innate immunity leading to increased infections and cancer [1]. The hallmark of aging cells is the shortening of the DNA telomeres. The thymus gland is of interest because it produces thymosin before birth and during childhood in order to generate T-lymphocytes and mature T-lymphocytes. At puberty, the thymus gland and thymosin production start to slowly disappear. By age 75, there is no thymus tissue present. Most T-cells are produced by puberty, and your peripheral T-cell pool loses function and replicative ability as you age. It is these age-related T cell changes and loss of thymic function that contribute greatly to the age-related decline of the immune system [3].

A Healthy Lifestyle Has a Healthy Immune System

There are many websites on the internet promoting supplements to boost your immune system. There is very little scientific data to support these claims. The Harvard Health page recommends: no smoking; decrease alcohol consumption; exercise regularly; eat fruits and vegetables; maintain a "healthy" weight; adequate sleep; avoid stress; wash your hands frequently; and cook meat adequately.

In this chapter, we have reviewed how a healthy lifestyle will build a healthy immune system. The essentials are summarized here and are covered in detail throughout this book.

1. A diet with adequate protein, carbohydrates, fat, and most importantly fiber—see chapter on fiber. A diet of unprocessed food grown in the ground or food that runs, flies, walks, or swims without antibiotics or preservatives. Healthy food usually does not come in a can or box—there are some exceptions.

2. Regular endurance and resistance exercises to the best of your ability. Minimum 30 minutes of cardiovascular HIIT exercises three times per week or more, and resistance training for each muscle group once a week.

3. People who have a viral syndrome or bacterial infection have increased metabolic demands for vitamins, minerals, and calories. Likewise, people who exercise regularly will have increased demands. In these situations, supplements are helpful to maintain adequate amounts of vitamins D, C, E; zinc, selenium, arginine, and glutamine.

4. Adequate sleep and stress avoidance.

5. Avoid alcohol as much as possible since alcohol is a bone marrow suppressant—it kills the cells of the immune system.

6. Stop smoking. Smoking causes lung damage. Your lungs are in constant contact with the outside environment and are a site of heightened immune activity.

7. A low-body-fat body—as low as you can comfortably go.

Is There a Supplement That Can Boost Your Immunity?—Thymosin Alpha 1

There is no level-1 data that can identify a supplement that will do this. There is one supplement that is very interesting. The thymus gland in children stimulates the production and maturation of T lymphocytes. The thymus gland disappears with age, and T-cell function declines. **Thymosin alpha 1 (Ta1)** is a hormone secreted by the thymus gland that modulates T-cell production and maturation. The rationale for the use of thymosin alpha 1 is to restore T-cell function in adults or patients with immune dysfunction. Thymosin alpha 1 had efficacy in a government-sponsored randomized trial in patients with severe sepsis [9]. Thymosin alpha 1 has shown benefit in human clinical studies in patients with bacterial infections, viral infections, hepatitis B and C, acquired immune deficiency syndromes, and many malignancies [10]. Ta1 is well tolerated and has an excellent safety profile. Ta1 is available by prescription only at many pharmacies in the USA and is not a controlled substance. You must discuss this with your physician.

CHAPTER 23
Evolution, Progress, Change

You Were Born to Exercise

We are Homo sapiens, and our species evolved from archaic species in the Middle Awash of Ethiopia, per objective fossil evidence. According to Rebecca Cann, the region where people have lived the longest should have the greatest genetic diversity—and Africa has the greatest genetic diversity.

Based on mitochondrial DNA evidence, we are all related to a woman who lived in Africa 100,000 to 200,000 years ago. The Middle Awash region of Ethiopia may be the place where people have lived the longest. Fossil evidence in the area reveals the presence of hominids (erect bipedal primates) who predate modern humans and are likely our immediate ancestors [1].

Early hominids were not the dominant species but rather were hunted as prey. What changes were necessary for modern humans to become the dominant species as we are today? A reasonable theory, based on fossil and anatomic evidence, is that the adaptation to long-distance running improved food scavenging, thus increasing brain size and the subsequent dominance of Homo sapiens—the human species.

Early hominids could walk, but their skeletons suggest that they could not run well. The early species were adapted to tree dwelling, with long toes and an appositional first foot digit (thumb). Modern toes are short, straight, and more energy-efficient for running. Modern human legs are longer relative to body mass, decreasing the energy expended while running. The modern human plantar arches and Achilles tendons provide sources of elastic, spring-like energy useful only when running.

Most animal species can run faster than humans, but most cannot run *farther*. Most medium to large mammals pant to prevent overheating while running. Modern humans sweat to prevent overheating, and this is done over a greater body surface area and is thus more efficient.

The theory of persistence hunting is that modern humans used endurance running to drive animals into hyperthermia and thus could be more easily hunted [2].

Thus, all modern humans have a body uniquely adapted over thousands of years to endurance exercise. What your body is unable to do is adapt to a sedentary, modern lifestyle. Therefore, more people today are suffering from chronic metabolic diseases.

According to the National Institute on Aging, there has been a dramatic increase in average life expectancy during the 20th century. Most babies born in 1900 did not live past the age of 50. **Life expectancy at birth in the U.S. (as of 2012) now exceeds 78 years.**

The real question is, **are we living *better* lives?** The National Center for Biological Technology Information states, "The leading risk factors related to disability life years were dietary risks, tobacco smoking, high body mass index, high blood pressure, high fasting plasma glucose, physical inactivity, and alcohol use." In simple terms, **metabolic disabilities in the U.S. comprise a larger share of life expectancy. We are not adapting well to our longer lives,**

and the problem is not simply aging but rather personal lifestyle choices.

James Fries made this very clear in his classic 50-year study of 1,741 people at the University of Pennsylvania [3]. Cumulative lifetime disability was four times greater in those who smoked, were obese, and did not exercise than in those who did not smoke, were lean, and exercised.

According to Fries, despite the current reduction in smoking today, there is still an increase in obesity in the U.S., and the percentage of people who exercise has remained stable. **We, as a nation, could be healthier if more of us exercised and ate an intelligent diet.**

Not all scientists and physicians agree that diet and exercise alone will make us healthier. Questions regarding exactly how caloric restriction prolongs longevity remain unanswered.

We will never be able to do a controlled prospective long-term study of caloric restrictions in humans because it would be considered unethical. We can study this subject in primates and lesser species only.

There has only been one such prospective controlled primate study completed, done at the University of Wisconsin from 1989 to 2009. This study clearly showed that **calorie restriction increased longevity by 56.2% [4]. How to explain this is still being debated and studied.**

There are negative effects of caloric restriction, which depend on the degree of starvation. During World War II, a group of lean men restricted their calorie intake by 45% for six months and ate mostly carbohydrates [5]. This starvation resulted in many positive metabolic changes—decreased body fat, lower blood pressure, lower serum cholesterol, lower resting heart rate, and a lower daily caloric resting expenditure (REE). This caloric restriction also had negative effects—anemia, swollen lower extremities due to lower serum proteins, muscle weakness, lethargy, and depression. These negative effects were also caused by the lack of protein and fat in this unhealthy, predominantly carbohydrate (90%) diet. The question remains, what caused the beneficial effects?

We have already discussed reactive oxygen species (ROS), also called free radicals. In the presence of high blood glucose/sugar levels—such as when overeating—mitochondria in all cells become less efficient and must work harder. These stressed mitochondria produce more ROS. The increased ROS then cause more damage to our DNA and kill more cells.

In the presence of calorie restriction and low blood glucose levels, our mitochondria work less, are more efficient, and produce less ROS. Less ROS means there is less DNA damage, fewer cells are killed, and we live longer.

Today, there is great interest in finding drugs or supplements that will prolong life span and emulate in humans the same effects of calorie restriction but *without* the calorie restriction. Calorie restriction activates certain genes (SIR2 and PNC1). These genes are the targets of this new area of drug research [6].

To date, no drug or supplement has been found that mimics the beneficial effects of calorie restriction. What does this mean to you? **It means that you still need to exercise and diet intelligently in order to have a healthy lifestyle.**

Modern Society and Hunter-Gatherers

Hunter-gatherers obtain their food by hunting wild animals and gathering wild plants. For most of human history, hunting and gathering were how we obtained our food. Farming and domestication of animals eventually replaced hunting and gathering in nearly all parts of the world. Today, just a small number of hunter-gatherers remain, and it is instructive to compare the health of modern society to that of modern hunter-gatherers.

Some hunger-gatherers can be found in the Americas, Africa, and Asia. If we compare a simple health marker—such as blood pressure—it appears that **modern hunter-gatherers are healthier than our modern industrialized population.**

Progress is the Root of All Evil— How Our Modern Lifestyle Changed Our Health

In 1956, my mother took me to see the play *Li'l Abner*. This musical, based on the comic strip *Li'l Abner*, contains a song called "Progress is the Root of All Evil." I didn't understand this refrain when I was 12 years old, but now, many years later, I understand what Johnny Mercer was saying.

With regard to our bodies and health, modern society has given us many new problems. Thousands of years ago, when hunter-gatherers became sedentary farmers, they were able to grow more food and domesticate farm animals. This abundance of calories allowed women to increase their birth rate. The average birth rate of sedentary farmers is estimated to be double that of hunter-gatherers [7]. Farm children became farmers as well, and populations grew, as did the abundance of food, leading to cities, free time, art, and culture.

Sedentary farmers tend to grow mostly carbohydrates (corn in some cultures), leading to a diet higher in carbohydrates than in the diets of hunter-gatherers. The Industrial Revolution of 1760 to 1840 essentially **replaced the use of human muscle with machines.** Our society changed, our diet changed to include more carbohydrates, and we used and needed less muscle. Most people will continue to drive their cars to work and use elevators. Few will choose to walk. However, **our metabolism remains unchanged, and this is the problem.**

Modern society has more metabolic health problems than did our ancient ancestors, as we demonstrated above—hypertension, diabetes, heart disease, and stroke—all owing to our unhealthy modern lifestyle. **We still have basically the same type of body as did our ancient hunter-gatherer ancestors, but we live in a culture with dangerous food options and fewer requirements for muscular strength.**

The best we can do is to understand our body and give our body the lifestyle it needs in order to remain healthy in these dangerous modern times.

Blood Pressure

One important measure of your overall health is your blood pressure (BP), and we can use this measure to compare relative health between our modern society and contemporary hunter-gatherers.

The heart pumps blood into the arteries (blood vessels that convey blood to all parts of the body). When the heart muscle (left ventricle) contracts, the pressure created to push blood out into the arteries is the systolic—first number of a blood pressure reading (measured in millimeters of mercury). Normal systolic blood pressure is below 120.

When your heart muscle relaxes between beats, the pressure maintained in your arteries is the diastolic blood pressure. A normal diastolic blood pressure is below 80.

Blood pressure is reported using both the systolic and diastolic numbers 120/80. An elevated blood pressure, such as 145/95, is called hypertension. In general, the lower your blood pressure, the longer you will live.

Men and women with hypertension have a shorter life expectancy and a higher risk of coronary artery disease, myocardial infarction, and stroke [8].

In one study, normotensive men and women survive 7.2 years longer without cardiovascular disease compared to hypertensive men and women. Compared to hypertensives, total life expectancy was longer for both normotensive men and women. Increased blood pressure in adulthood is associated with reduction in life expectancy.

Blood pressure readings of modern hunter-gatherers are well below the modern industrialized average of <120/<80—Bushmen at 108/63, Yanomamo at 104/65, Xingu at 107/68, and Kitava at 113/71. In addition, blood pressure does not increase with age as it does in North Americans.

Other health marker improvements in the hunter-gatherers include increased insulin sensitivity, lower plasma insulin levels, lower leptin levels, lower BMI, smaller waist size, and lower skinfold measurements. **It appears that our modern lifestyle has made our bodies less healthy.**

Why We Continue to Eat Bad Food

As a society, we continue to eat bad food because we are not knowledgeable about food—we are marketed about our food. We are addicted to sugar, and we drink too much alcohol. We don't use the knowledge that's outlined in this book.

Here are **FOUR** additional reasons we make bad food choices:

The first is that the obesity epidemic in this country has been aided by the low cost of high glucose-containing carbohydrates. These foods (soybeans and corn) are inexpensive because their production and storage is subsidized by the U.S. government in the Farm Bill. For the past 50 years, U.S. farm policy has been directed towards driving down the price of farmed storable carbohydrates (again, corn and soybeans).

At the same time, the cost of growing fruits and vegetables has increased, as has their retail price. Low costs cause the food industry to use more of these unhealthy commodities. High-fructose corn syrup is now commonly added to many foods (*processed* foods).

In summary, the food industry has a huge financial incentive to make food with high-glycemic carbohydrates.

The second reason we eat bad food is due to marketing. Marketing is defined as, whatever it takes to make you buy a specific product.

One of the most useful marketing techniques is to aim marketing messages at children, who then nag their parents to buy this or that product. Then the child may continue to buy that product well into adulthood.

The food industry spends over $1.6 billion dollars in marketing food to children [HBO documentary series *The Weight of the Nation*, May 2012.] Most of these products are processed foods which are high in calories and sugar and often lead to obesity.

Every month, approximately 90% of American children between the ages of three and nine years visit a McDonald's. [*Fast Food Nation*, Schlosser E, Mariner Books, Houghton Mifflin Harcourt, 2012.] Is it a coincidence that McDonalds operates over 8,000 restaurant playgrounds [10]?

Fast food chains profit when children drink soda because soda has the highest profit margin. Today, McDonald's sells more

Coca-Cola than anyone else in the world. A medium Coke that sells for $1.29 contains roughly 9 cents' worth of syrup [10].

The third reason we continue to eat poorly is the belief that *labels do not lie*. Marketing companies have created labels using a selection of words that make us believe we are eating healthy food when in fact we are not.

Whole grain refers to a cereal product containing the germ endosperm and bran and is thus *not* refined or man-made. Yet the stamp *whole grain* from the Whole Grains Council means the product must contain only 8 grams of whole grain per 30 grams of product and thus is mostly *not* comprised of whole grains. The label stating "Made With Whole Grain" actually may mean that only a tiny amount of whole grain is present.

The label *Heart Healthy*, sold by the American Heart Association for use on foods, refers to the fat and salt content of a product but *not* the sugar content. Thus, the real cause of heart disease is not even accounted for.

The term "all natural" really should be labeled "stay away!" The USDA does not define foods labeled "all natural" as any different than those labeled "natural". Foods with this labeling are usually not any different than *natural* foods and may not be regulated as they are not defined by the USDA. Foods labeled "natural," according to the USDA definition, do not contain artificial ingredients or preservatives, and the ingredients are only minimally processed. However, they may contain antibiotics, growth hormones, and other similar chemicals. People often confuse natural with organic, but they are not the same.

The fourth reason we eat poorly is that much of our food is ultra-processed, as noted in chapter 9. Ultra-processed food increases appetite, calorie intake, and causes insulin-resistant cells.

CHAPTER 24
Plant-Based Diet?

Today's popular culture is enthusiastic about a diet that is plant based. Many celebrities are now vegetarians—Jennifer Lopez, Jessica Simpson, Jay-Z, Beyonce, Woody Harrelson, Ellen DeGeneres, Bill Clinton, Brad Pitt, Alec Baldwin, Miley Cyrus, Demi Moore, Stevie Wonder, and many more. Is there any scientific reason to follow a plant-based diet?

Consumer Reports author Rachel Meltzer Warren wrote an article "The Benefits of a Plant-Based Diet," and referred to the following studies: JAMA study of 70,000 people; preliminary study of 450,000 adults with a 70% plant-based diet had 20% lower risk of dying from heart disease or stroke; Harvard study of 120,000 people for 30 years died younger if ate meat; American Journal of Cardiology plant-based diet decreased total cholesterol and LDL. In addition, there were testimonials from Robert Ostfeld M.D., Reed Mangels Ph.D., and Sharon Palmer R.D.N.

The JAMA study evaluated 73,308 Seventh-day Adventists [1].

This population does not smoke or drink and is partly vegetarian, allowing eggs and dairy. In this study, only the male vegetarians lived longer than the male non-vegetarians. Women were unaffected. A flaw in this study was the control group of non-vegetarians who lived on the East Coast of the USA, where the incidence of heart attack mortality was 38% higher than the vegetarians who lived on the West Coast. In addition, the non-vegetarians were not all non-smokers and non-drinkers, and this variable was not well-controlled. Another design flaw was that this study was designed by, supported by, and evaluated by West Coast Seventh-Day Adventists whose bias favored strict adherence to their religion. Currently, the European study of 450,000 adults has not been published. The above Harvard study was data from the Nurse's Health Study II, combined with other data that concluded eating an additional 3 ounces of red meat per day was associated with a 12% increased risk of dying. There was not a simple dose response—the more meat, the greater risk—as one would predict. It was only the very high meat eaters that had the increased risk. These people were least likely to exercise, most likely to be obese, and most likely to smoke. The Harvard study did not control these important variables. Today, total cholesterol and total LDL are not accurate measures of cardiac risk. Total cholesterol includes both HDL and LDL, and elevated HDL is a marker of health. Total LDL is a mixture of small particle and large particle LDL. You can have a low total LDL, which is mostly small particles and can be very unhealthy because the small particle LDL is the most destructive lipid element, and no epidemiological studies comparing diets have measured small particle LDL.

The most quoted study favoring a plant-based diet to prevent many diseases is the China Study published in book form by T. Colin Campbell Ph.D., Thomas Campbell, and Jacob Gould Schurman. This large epidemiological study of 65 counties in China are observations and opinions without experimental design. There are no examples of a population of vegetarians in China. Campbell's hypothesis is that eating animal protein causes cancer and many other diseases. Campbell's methods were not direct measures of actual food intake but indirect measures from food composition tables. The data came from the Chinese government.

A 2017 meta-analysis of 29 studies has concluded that consuming dietary dairy fat has no negative effects on all-cause mortality or mortality from cardiovascular disease (CVD) and coronary heart disease (CHD). This includes fats of all types [2].

The dietary opinions of experts are level-4 data and very controversial. The expert testimonials are sincere because these physicians placed patients on plant-based diets and watched them improve. The one intervention that always prolongs longevity in every species tested is a reduction in calories [3]. How you choose to do this is always your choice. Low calories can be achieved with a vegetable-based diet as well as a diet containing animal protein and fat. Remember that there are no essential carbohydrates—only essential proteins and essential fats.

This fact is without question—when I place my patients on a non-vegetarian, low-calorie diet, they universally improve, and many no longer need their prescription medication for hypertension, hyperlipidemia, and type 2 diabetes.

In summary, to live a long, healthy life, stay educated, lean and exercise—do not follow the popular culture.

CHAPTER 25
Telomeres and Longevity and Senescent Cells

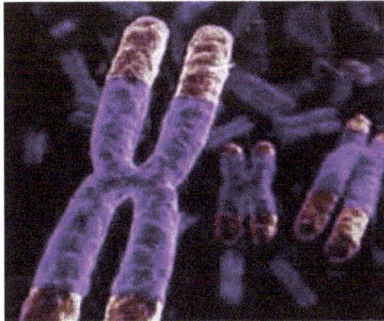

Many theories have been proposed to explain why people age. Most theories blame aging on damage to your DNA (deoxyribonucleic acid). Before you can understand the theories regarding aging and longevity, we must define our terms. The cells in your body contain your genetic information in the form of 23 pairs of chromosomes. Each cell contains the same genetic information—the same 23 chromosomes. This is your DNA. Each chromosome is made up of sequences of four nucleic acids—adenine, guanine, thymine, and cytosine. You are a multicellular animal that requires the cells in your body (somatic cells) to divide in order for you to grow, maintain, and repair your body. The cells that produce eggs and sperm are not included in this discussion. During cell division (mitosis) one cell divides into two daughter cells, each containing the same 23 pairs of chromosomes. However, if this statement were completely true, you could possibly live forever. During chromosome replication in dividing cells (mitosis), the enzymes (chemicals that cause reactions) that duplicate the DNA cannot duplicate the DNA all the way to the end of the chromosome. When a somatic cell divides, the end of the chromosome—the telomere—is shortened, resulting in a small loss of DNA.

THE ENDS OF THE CHROMOSOMES ARE THE TELO-MERES.IN EVERY SOMATIC CELL DIVISION, SOME DNA IS LOST.

The length of one type of cell telomere—your peripheral blood lymphocytes—can be easily measured by a simple blood test. The length of these telomeres is approximately 8,000 base pairs in newborns; approximately 3,000 base pairs in average adults; and down to 1,500 base pairs in the elderly. Remember, we are measuring only the end of the chromosome since the entire chromosome has approximately 150 million base pairs. Each time a cell divides, it loses between 30 to 200 base pairs. On average, a cell can divide 50 to 70 times before it dies. Cell death can be attributed to this loss of DNA, and theoretically this is the aging process [1]. Telomere length can be used as an objective marker for aging and longevity [2]. In this setting, telomere length (TL) is similar for men and women and similar for their children. Thus, a heritable link is present. **TL does decrease with age.** TL is associated with more years of healthy life but not overall survival [3]. **Relative telomere length is a marker for a healthy lifestyle within a given individual.** One path toward longer telomeres is through exercise. TL is preserved in healthy older adults who perform vigorous aerobic exercise and is positively related to maximal aerobic exercise capacity [4]. This may represent a novel molecular mechanism underlying the anti-aging effects of maintaining high aerobic capacity. In another study of 70 males and females 50 to 70 years of age, a moderate physical activity level over the past 5 years or longer was significantly associated with telomere length [5].

240

Acute exercise may not be a strong enough stimulus to cause short-term changes to telomere length. The telomere length data from the Ludlow study indicates that a very low level of exercise and an extremely high level of exercise are associated with shorter telomere length compared with moderate levels of exercise over a long period of time. Telomeres are also particularly susceptible to free radicals that are thought to be major contributors to the aging process [6, 7]. Once telomeres shorten to a critical length, the cell dies [8]. Telomeres can be elongated by the enzyme telomerase [9], which is repressed in most normal adult somatic tissues because telomerase activation is necessary for cancer cells to maintain telomeres over multiple rounds of cell division [Forsyth et al. 2002]. Thus, telomere shortening is thought to act as both an anti-cancer mechanism and contribute to the aging process [10]. **It appears that individual TL during one's lifetime could provide a measure of that individual's healthy lifestyle.**

Senescent Cells

Another theory of aging involves the idea that as your body ages, it accumulates cells that do not divide and do not die—senescent cells. Senescent cells increase in our tissues as we age [11]. Cellular senescence is caused by a variety of events leading to the idea that there are different types of senescent cells [12]. Senescence can be caused by telomere shortening, DNA damage by reactive oxygen species, activation of genes that stop cell division, exposure to interferon-b, exposure to inflammatory cytokines, methylation, and other inhibitors. Whenever damaged cells expose DNA, a group of survival genes are activated to prevent these damaged and potentially oncogenic cells from dividing. The theory is that these cells, if they divide, would be malignant. Some of these non-dividing cells—senescent cells—produce cytokines/molecules that can be inflammatory or anti-inflammatory, neoplastic or anti-neoplastic. Senescent cells can be pathologic and cause age-related diseases [13]. The beneficial effects of exercise on health have been reviewed in chapter 11 and are irrefutable. The exact beneficial cellular mechanisms that exercise produces are not completely known. In general, exercise overcomes the harmful effect of excess calories. Exercise also prevents cellular senescence in visceral body fat [14]. This is a new and important finding since senescent cells are implicated in the development of aging, and their removal increases lifespan [13].

Senescent Cell Formation

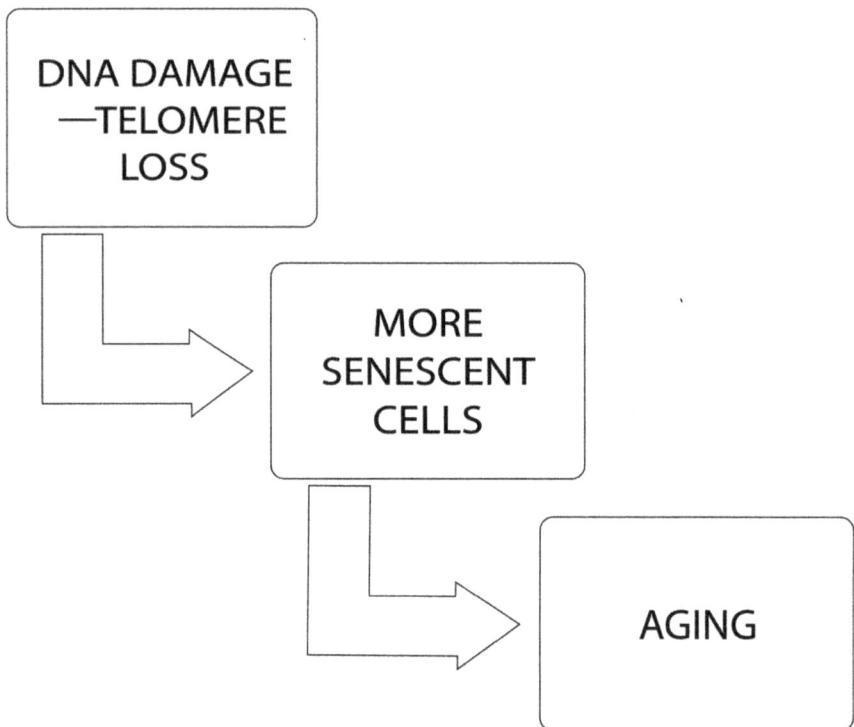

DNA DAMAGE —TELOMERE LOSS

MORE SENESCENT CELLS

AGING

CHAPTER 26
Anti-Aging

The Telomere Shortening Theory of aging is important because it provides objective data about longevity and human behavior.

In the Telomere Shortening Theory, whenever a somatic cell divides, some DNA is lost. At some point, enough DNA is lost that the cell dies. Cell death is synonymous with aging, and telomere length shortens with age. If we assume that in a given individual Telomere length determines relative longevity, we should find things that preserve or lengthen Telomeres and counter the aging process.

Sex Hormones

In patients with abnormally short telomeres (diseases with mutations in the genes that repair and maintain telomeres), the drug danazol led to telomere elongation in both male and female patients [1]. Danazol is a weak androgen, or male sex hormone, and a weak anabolic steroid. Normal lymphocytes (white blood cells), when exposed to androgens or estrogen, increase the production of telomerase, which lengthens telomeres. The estrogen blocker and pseudo-estrogen tamoxifen blocks this activity for both androgens and estrogens. Letrazol, an aromatase inhibitor, blocked only estrogen from increasing telomerase, while the androgen receptor blocker Futamide had no effect [2]. Post-menopausal women on hormone replacement therapy have longer telomeres than post-menopausal women not on therapy [3].

Based upon the above data, it is reasonable to conclude that normal sex hormone levels and supplemented sex hormone levels to achieve normal levels are beneficial in regard to telomere preservation. The corollary is that low sex hormone levels are not beneficial.

Smoking and Obesity

The telomeres of obese women are significantly shorter than non-obese women, found in a study of 1,122 patients ages 18 to 76 years. In addition, this same study found a dose-dependent relationship between cigarette smoking and telomere length. For each pack of cigarettes smoked, a woman would lose five base pairs of telomere length [4] **Based upon this study, a lower body weight and no smoking benefit telomere length.** An interesting aside is that smoking causes skin wrinkles, a sign of aging [16].

Polycyclic Aromatic Hydrocarbons

Polycyclic aromatic hydrocarbons (PCAH) are known carcinogens and cause telomere shortening in a dose response fashion [5]. Polycyclic aromatic hydrocarbons are found as air pollutants in many workplace settings—coke ovens, coal tar production, asphalt production, smokehouses, and trash incinerators. They are also present in cigarette smoke, wood smoke, vehicle exhaust, and agricultural product fires. PCAHs are present in foods—burned meat, contaminated cereals, and processed or pickled foods. **Based upon this data, breathe clean air, and do not eat burned or processed foods.**

Life Stress

Chronic stress as defined in premenopausal mothers of chronically ill children have shorter telomeres when compared to an aged match control group of mothers with healthy children [6, 7]. **Avoid stress.**

Exercise

Endurance athletes, both young and old men and women, show an increase in telomere stabilizing proteins and longer telomeres than a similar population of non-endurance athletes [7]. The differences were striking and explain the benefits of exercise in regard to preventing endothelial cell pathology and preventing age-related diseases.

Exercise is essential for telomere health. In addition, exercise prevents the development of senescent cells.

Alcohol

A study of telomere length in alcoholic patients versus patients who did not drink alcohol presented at the Denver meeting of the Research Society on Alcoholism clearly showed that alcohol decreases telomere length [8]. Drinking makes you older at the cellular level. **Alcohol is bad.**

Processed Meats

A population of 2,846 American Indians were studied in regard to telomere length and consumption of red meat and processed meat. The study group was adjusted in regard to age, sex, smoking, alcohol, exercise, and education. Telomere length was significantly lower in those who ate processed meat [9].

Vitamin D

Serum vitamin D levels were measured in 2,160 women aged 18-79 years. Higher vitamin D levels were correlated with greater telomere length [10, 11].

Mutant Mitochondrial Free Radical Theories Oxidative Stress

The mutant mitochondrial and free radical theories of aging propose that free radicals—molecules that donate electrons—cause genetic defects or DNA mutations that can kill cells. The cell damage caused by oxygen-containing free radicals in this sequence of events is called oxidative stress. Mitochondria are especially vulnerable. Oxidative stress is a normal product in all living cells. The body produces anti-oxidants to counter free radicals. Despite the body's response, oxidative stress can cause telomere dysfunction and shortening [11]. Oxidative stress has been implicated in many disease states, including cancers, autoimmune diseases, and immune deficiencies [12].

Supplements That May Prolong Your Life

Metformin

Metformin is an FDA-approved drug for the treatment of type 2 diabetes. Metformin lowers blood sugar levels, increases insulin sensitivity in muscle cells, and decreases the amount of sugar produced in the liver. In animal and in vitro studies, Metformin improves age-related conditions by decreasing inflammation, oxidative damage, cell senescence and apoptosis. Metformin targets multiple age-related conditions in addition to improving type 2 diabetes.

Specifically, Metformin has been shown to have a beneficial effect upon the receptors for insulin, cytokines, IGF-1, and adiponectin. Metformin inhibits inflammatory pathways, activates AMPK, and decreases mTOR, all of which are associated with longevity. The mechanisms by which Metformin induces senescent cell removal, decreases inflammation, and prolongs cellular survival are unclear. Currently, human data is pending, and the specific pathways that prolong longevity are unclear [13]. Unfortunately, metformin will lower testosterone levels [16].

Sirtuins—NAD—Senescent Cells

Calorie restriction is the only proven method to counter the aging process. A possible mechanism underlying the benefit of calorie restriction is to increase the production of Sir2 proteins inside cells. As animals and humans age, intercellular NAD decreases. NAD (nicotinamide adenine dinucleotide) is a co-enzyme that enables our mitochondria to turn our foods into usable intracellular energy. Decreased NAD reduces sirtuins, and these changes disrupt the communication between the cell nucleus and mitochondria and also between the hypothalamus and your body fat. These changes cause the functional decline that occurs with aging. NAD supplementation is currently being studied in human subjects [14].

Aging is molecular and cellular decline that decreases tissue function over time, leading to disease and death. The features of health include telomere length, accurate cellular division, stable protein (hormones, peptides, ligands) communication, and mitochondrial integrity.

All living species age at different rates. All living cells accumulate molecular damage that leads to defective mitochondria, impaired intracellular communication, and senescent cells. Environmental factors—epigenetics—stress the cells, and healthy aging is the ability of cells to respond effectively to these epigenetic stress factors. Calorie restriction is the single most effective way to prolong longevity and delay aging [17].

In summary, an anti-aging lifestyle requires calorie restriction, no smoking, lower emotional stress, aerobic exercise, vitamin D, hormone replacement or supplements, a diet free from alcohol and processed meats, a body that is not obese, and clean air. There is no clear evidence that taking an antioxidant is helpful [15].

Adult longevity appears dependent on the metabolic pathways that shut down cell division and muscle development and increase cellular efficiency. Please refer to chapter 19.

CHAPTER 27
Peptide Therapy

A peptide is made of two or more linked amino acids. What a specific peptide does is determined by its length and amino acid sequence. Peptides have many roles to play in your body since they can transport molecules into cells, act as hormones to change cell function, and act as neurotransmitters. A protein is a peptide with at least 50 amino acids. Hormones carry messages from one cell to another and may be peptides, proteins, or glycoproteins (carbohydrate protein complex). To understand how peptides may be helpful, you must understand how your body works.

The pituitary gland at the base of the brain controls the production of many hormones—ACTH stimulates the adrenal glands to produce hormones; FSH and LH stimulate the female ovaries and the male testes; GH maintains growth in children and muscle, bone and fat distribution in adults; prolactin stimulates breast milk production; TSH stimulates the thyroid gland; ADH stimulates the kidneys to retain water; and oxytocin stimulates the uterus during childbirth and helps with breast milk production. Adults with growth hormone (GH) deficiency have increased body fat, decreased muscle mass, decreased bone density, and a lower capacity to exercise. GH levels decrease as you
1 age. Is this what makes people age? Can GH supplements improve the health of the elderly?

Growth Hormone

Growth hormone (GH) acts on the liver to produce IGF-1, or Insulin-like Growth Factor one. IGF-1 is responsible for the growth-promoting effect of GH, and the IGF-1 blood level is a measure of GH production. GH itself is difficult to measure directly since it has a very short half-life. A low level of growth hormone in a child or adult can occur, and this is called growth hormone deficiency—GHD. In childhood GHD, the cause is usually unknown. In adults, the cause is usually a pituitary tumor, radiation, or head trauma. The signs of GHD in children include short stature, delayed physical maturation, and poor muscular development. In adults, GHD causes reduced muscle mass, low bone density, elevated LDL, reduced energy, and increased body fat. The FDA has approved the use of human growth hormone to treat well documented cases of GHD. The diagnosis requires multiple measures, including body measurements, blood level of IGF-1, and a provocative test giving a GH stimulant intravenously, followed by serial blood tests for IGF-1. This test may take several hours to perform.

Between ages 20 and 60, IGF-1 levels may decrease by 90%. This may be termed the normal aging process. **I would call this an unhealthy metabolic state that should be treated with diet and exercise first.** During this period, body fat increases and muscle mass decreases. Giving GH to healthy men between ages 60 and 81 for six or twelve months, whose IGF-1 levels were below 350 IU/liter, resulted in increased bone density and lean body mass—less fat and more muscle on a percentage basis [1]. **It was as if ten to twenty years of aging were apparently reversed with GH.**

One important aspect of GH not included in the above study is the effect of exercise on GH. Exercise raises GH and causes similar benefits. No long-term studies with GH have been performed, and the effect of GH on the incidence of cancer remains unstudied in humans and is a serious concern. There has been little additional GH scientific data since 1990. Today, GH is included in the 1990 Anabolic Steroids Control Act. **The use of GH other than the treatment of the disease GHD is criminalized as a five-year felony under the penalties chapter of the Food, Drug, and Cosmetics Act of the FDA. GH remains as the only FDA-approved drug that is a felony for off-label use.** In my opinion, this law is based upon level-4 recommendations and not upon scientific data. Physicians must obey the law.

Sermorelin

Sermorelin is a growth hormone-releasing peptide normally produced by the brain. Administration of Sermorelin causes the pituitary gland to produce growth hormone and may be a better alternative than administering GH—Sermorelin can be administered off-label and is not a controlled substance. Giving GH will diminish the natural pituitary production of GH, while giving Sermorelin increases the pituitary production of GH [2]. Giving Sermorelin raises GH levels in a normal, physiologic setting. There are no long-term studies in adults.

Other Growth Hormone-Releasing Peptides

Other interesting peptides were discovered by their ability to restore cardiac cell function in the experimental setting of ischemia and reperfusion [1]. Some of these new peptides were more beneficial than GH in this experimental setting. In this setting, ghrelin was discovered. Ghrelin is a 28-amino-acid peptide/hormone that is secreted by gastric cells and induces hunger. Ghrelin releases GH and is protective for many different cell populations, including heart muscle cells. GHRP-6 is a potent peptide that increases GH release by the pituitary gland. This GH stimulus is potentiated by insulin and diminished by the consumption of carbohydrates and/or fat. GHRP-2 is a GH-releasing peptide that also stimulates the release of ghrelin. CJC-1295 markedly increases GH and IGF-1 blood levels because it has a half-life of six to eight days. With CJC-1295, GH levels can increase up to ten times and remain elevated for six days [2].

In summary, your IGF-1 level is an important measure of your GH production and controls your body composition. Exercise increases growth hormone production. This is another reason to include exercise in your lifestyle.

CHAPTER 28
Summary: How to Optimize Your Body—13 Steps

1. Optimize Your Weight: In your web browser, visit Mayo Clinic's calorie calculator: (www.mayoclinic.org/healthy-lifestyle/nutrition-and-healthy-eating/in-depth/calorie-calculator/itt-20084939). Calculate how many calories you need every day. If you wish to decrease body fat, subtract 300 to 500 calories from your daily calorie number. Use the resulting number as an approximation of your daily caloric limit in order to target one pound of weight loss per week. If you wish to gain weight, increase your calculated calorie needs by 300 to 500 calories.

2. Calculate your protein needs based on your weight with 1 gram of protein per pound of body weight. This will provide your daily protein and fat. If you wish to gain weight, calculate your protein needs at 2 grams of protein per pound of body weight.

3. Calculate the calorie content of your protein meals by weighing your food on a food scale or using package labels. Daily diet calories minus protein and fat calories equals carbohydrate calories. This resulting number is the number of calories you should obtain from intermediate glycemic carbohydrates.

4. Select healthy foods as described in this book. Eat all the green vegetables and salads that you can—the more fiber, the better; these calories do not count. No alcohol.

5. Weigh yourself frequently, and keep a written or electronic journal. Measure your waist size once a month. If possible, obtain a DEXA scan yearly to truly know your body composition.

6. Do 30 to 40 minutes of vigorous cardiovascular exercise three times per week—treadmill, elliptical, bike, running, jogging, swimming. Exercise on the days you don't do weight training until you can't talk.

7. Resistance—train each muscle group once a week—pushing on Monday, legs on Wednesday, pulling on Friday, with a rest day in between. Your muscles grow during these rest periods. Drink whey protein during or after these resistance exercises.

8. Sleep and allow your body to recover. Rest, without engaging in any exercise, one or two days per week. Do not eat after your evening meal until breakfast. If you can, fast 12 hours to increase autophagy by eating only when it is daylight.

9. Take supplements and hormone replacement as needed. The minimum supplements include a multivitamin, vitamin D3, and fish or krill oil. Obtain blood tests—t3, free t3, t4, tsh, testosterone free and total, estradiol, CBC, complete metabolic profile, lipid profile, CRP and homocysteine. Median normal to upper normal hormone levels are optimal for vitality. Vitality and longevity require balance.

10. Expect your body to change slowly. You must change your diet and exercise program as your body changes in order to continue to improve slowly. It's a lifestyle, a path without end, a race won by the turtle.

11. There are only three things that will increase your metabolic rate and decrease your appetite—a medical weight loss pill, exercise, and fat in the diet. If obese, do all three. Otherwise, do the last two.

12. Say, "Show me the data!" to anyone giving health advice. Keep an open mind, and stay up-to-date regarding scientific advances. Resistance exercise is required for vitality. Cardiovascular exercise is required for longevity. Scientists still cannot fully explain why calorie restriction increases lifespan.

13. When you achieve your goals and feel good and your weight is stable, you have achieved your optimal body. No two people are alike, and you are your only competition.

CHAPTER 29
The Authors

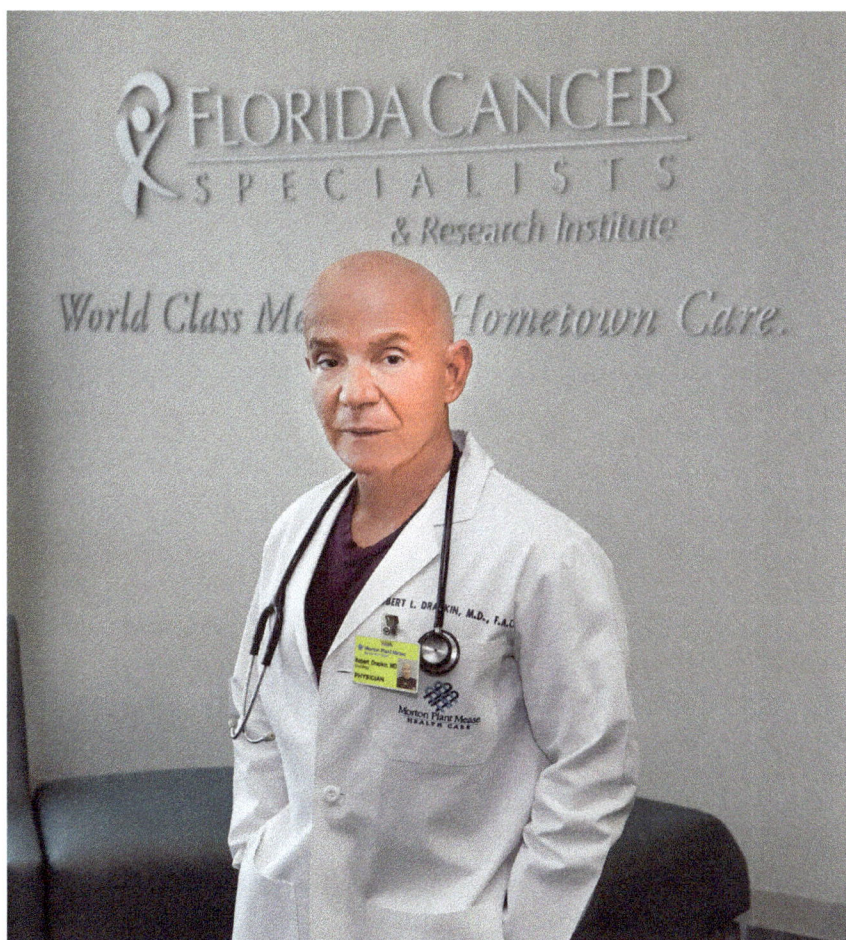

Robert Drapkin, MD, FACP

Robert Drapkin, MD, FACP

I am the son of a poor boy born in the town of Polotsk, Belarus around 1900. My dad lifted himself out of poverty with sheer determination and hard work so that he could attend medical school at the University of Bern, Switzerland. He became a general practitioner of medicine (MD) in Albany, New York and raised me, his only son. I was predestined to go to medical school; it was expected, and there were no other options in my life in Albany.

I look back with appreciation of my dad's guidance. I accepted early admission at Wayne State Medical School in Detroit, Michigan. I wanted to get away from New York State, where my dad had some influence.

In 1967, Wayne State was the only medical school in Detroit, and the clinical experience was intense. Every howling ambulance brought me a new problem to solve.

I did my internship and residency at the University of Illinois in Chicago—another trauma hospital with an active emergency room. I lived and breathed medicine. It was my entire life, and I loved it.

I became the Chief Resident and Instructor in Medicine my last year in Chicago and then accepted a fellowship in Medical Oncology at Memorial Sloan Kettering in New York City. I enjoyed Oncology, as it was complicated and interesting internal medicine.

My next academic role was as a full-time attending and assistant professor at Roswell Park Memorial Institute in Buffalo, New York—a New York State-managed oncology center. I always felt more comfortable at the bedside than in the laboratory, and I subsequently moved to the west coast of Florida in 1979, where the incidence of cancer was high and the oncology resources were few.

In summary, I've been an MD since 1971. I've been taking care of sick folks in an academic setting and in private practice for over 45 years. I learned almost everything I know from my patients.

Dr. Drapkin's Current Gym Training Schedule

I do 30 minutes of HIIT on an elliptical machine three times per week, and I exercise each muscle group to failure (weight lifting) one hour per day, four days per week, in a commercial gym. I recommend not building a home gym because part of your motivation comes from the other people in the gym. There is always much to learn from others, and new data is constantly forthcoming.

Before training, I eat a 510-calorie breakfast containing 30 grams of protein, 30 grams of carbohydrate, and approximately 30 grams of fat.

Before lifting any weights, I do myofascial release with a foam roller on the target muscles for that day as well as dynamic active and passive stretching with my trainer. I perform core-strengthening exercises.

I drink copious amounts of water throughout the hour of exercise. I sip branched-chain amino acids mixed with whey protein as well during my exercise.

Monday, I target the pushing muscles of the chest, shoulders, and triceps, followed by the abdominal muscles and ending with core exercises.

1. Chest press on a slight 30-degree incline bench with a barbell or dumbbells—three sets.

2. Chest press, as above, with a 45-degree incline or machine press—three sets (may do five-second negatives).

3. Military press—a 90-degree incline, as above, or machine—three sets (may do five-second negatives).

4. Triceps rope pull-downs and skull crushers with barbell—three sets.

5. Abdominal crunches with a 25-lb. dumbbell while resting on Bosu.

All sets are done to muscle failure. If it's possible to do 12 repetitions, the weight is increased with a target of six repetitions. For fewer than six repetitions, the weight is decreased. We aim for a one-minute rest between sets.

Wednesday is leg day:

1. Smith machine squats—four sets.

2. Inclined leg press—three sets followed by a drop set.

3. Leg extensions by machine.

4. Leg curls by machine.

5. Posterior chain back extensions.

Friday is back, trapezius and biceps day:

1. Pull-ups—three sets.

2. Horizontal cable row—three sets.

3. High cable row—three sets.

4. Mid-back inverted rows or dumbbell mid-back rows—three sets.

5. Trapezius Smith machine pull-ups—three sets.

6. Barbell biceps curls—four sets.

7. Abdominal crunches.

8. Core—planks on stability ball or foam roller and ball rollouts.

Saturday is optional—posterior chain leg and arms day:

1. Deadlifts.

2. Single-leg inclined leg press.

3. Balance exercises—running man on Bosu

4. Abdominal hanging leg pull-ups and Bosu crunches.

5. Core—planks on stability ball or foam roller and ball rollouts.

—Robert Louis Drapkin, MD, FACP

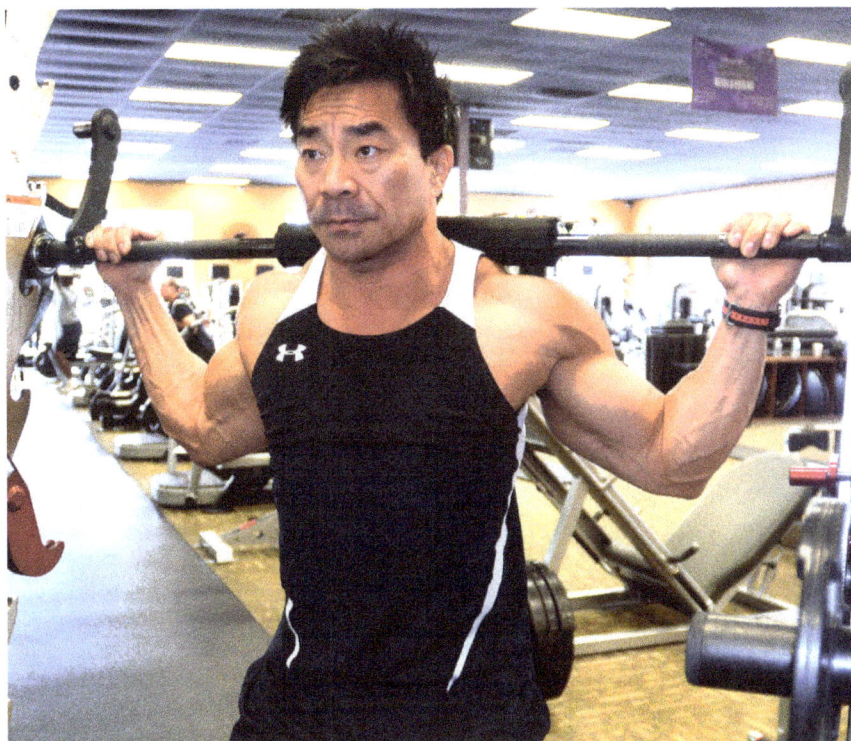

Donny H. Kim, PES, CPT-NASM

Donny H. Kim, PES, CPT-NASM, Master Trainer, was born in 1966 in Seoul, Korea. When his father's commercial trucking business came to a crashing halt in 1976, his family immigrated to the U.S. seeking a better life. Donny was ten years old at the time. He learned the alphabet and how to write his name in English just days before moving.

The language and cultural barriers were tough on the entire family, and especially for Donny's father. They first settled in Edgar, Nebraska from 1976 until 1978. It was a tiny town located in south-central Nebraska, mostly comprised of hard-working

German descendants. There were no other Korean families within a 50-mile radius. Looking back, Donny finds that this really helped them to become integrated into their new world. He still remembers his father's words: "Be a great representation of yourself, your family, and your nationality." He expressed that they needed to not just be better, but to be way better, in their new world. Donny's father also encouraged the family to excel in everything they did.

In 1978, the family moved to Michigan City, Indiana, where Donny's father had a distant relative. All through school, Donny thrived in academics and sports as well as leadership positions. He graduated with numerous high honors, highest varsity sport points, and served as the senior high school class president. He had ROTC scholarships available but decided to take the academic scholarship at Indiana University.

Donny did his undergraduate studies and attended law school at I.U. Bloomington. Starting in 1985, he oversaw the Student Athletic Center, and he entered his first bodybuilding competition, which he loved. Soon thereafter, he realized that a law career was his father's goal for him, and he found *his* passion in fitness and coaching. So after law school, he did everything he could find in the fitness business—presale, front desk, training, sales, and even general manager.

In late 1995, he relocated to Tampa Bay. Between 1995 and 2012, he became the top personal trainer and training manager for both Gold's Gym and Lifestyle Family Fitness. During this time, he won numerous bodybuilding titles, including Mr. Tampa Bay, Mr. Florida Natural, and World Superbody Runner-Up—Lightweight. He also earned the status of Professional Natural Bodybuilder.

Donny has modeled, acted, and more importantly served Tampa Bay as a fitness and nutrition expert. In 2012, he started Tampa Bay Fitness and continues to serve as its president.

Donny has an incredible home life with his beautiful wife, Angela, and his amazing son, Michael, who share his success, joy, and happiness. Put simply, he loves what he does. He has raving clients, he is respected by his peers, and he makes his living by helping others.

As of the time of this writing, Donny has been in the fitness industry for 30 years—and he's still happily exhausted every day. He hopes to continue to reach more and more people with his knowledge and passion.

Donny can be reached at donnykimfit@gmail.com or (727) 410-9210.

Bibliography

Chapter 1: The Most Important Thing

1. Kung HC, Hoyert DL, Xu JQ, Murphy SL. Deaths: national data for 2005. National Vital Statistics Reports 2008.

2. Wu SY, Green A. Projection of chronic illness prevalence and cost in nation. Santa Monica, CA: RAND Health; 2000.

3. Anderson G. Chronic conditions: making the case for ongoing care. Baltimore, MD: John Hopkins University; 2004.

4. Ursula E. Bauer, Peter A. Briss, Richard A. Goodman, Barbara A. Bowman. Prevention of chronic disease in the 21st century: elimination of the leading preventable causes of premature death and disability in the USA, The Lancet; 2014.

5. Age and Sex Patterns of Drug Prescribing in a Defined American Population. Wenjun Zhong, PhD, Hilal Maradit-Kremers, MD, MSc, Jennifer L. St. Sauver, PhD, MPH, Barbara P. Yawn, MD, MSc, Jon O. Ebbert, MD, Véronique L. Roger, MD, MPH, Debra J. Jacobson, MS, Michaela E. McGree, BS, Scott M. Brue, BS, Walter A. Rocca, MD, MPH.

Chapter 2: Americans Are Unhealthy—Sicker Than Any Other Industrialized Country

1. Mayo Clinic proceedings, ISSN: 1942-5546, Vol: 91, Issue: 4, Page: 432-42; 2016; Healthy Lifestyle Characteristics and Their Joint Association With Cardiovascular Disease Biomarkers in US Adults; Paul D. Loprinzi, Adam Branscum, PhD, June Hanks, PhD, DPT, PT, Ellen Smit, PhD.

2. Psychiatr Clin North Am. 2011 Dec; 34(4): 717–732. 10.1016/j.psc.2011.08.005 OBESITY: OVERVIEW OF AN EPIDEMIC Nia Mitchell, MD, Vicki Catenacci, MD, Holly R. Wyatt, MD, and James O. Hill, PhD.

3. The Lancet Vol 366, 5-11 November, p1640-1649, Obesity and the risk of myocardial infarction in 27,000 participants from 52 countries: a case-control study Salim Yusef et al.

4. The Lancet Vol 389, April 1, 2017 1323. Future life expectancy in 35 industrialised countries: projections with a Bayesian model ensemble. Vasilis Kontis, James E. Bennett, Colin D. Mathers, Guangquan Li, Kyle Foreman, Majid Ezzati.

5. U.S. Health in International Perspective: Shorter Lives, Poorer Health; National Research Council (US); Institute of Medicine SH Woolf and L Aron.

6. National Vital Statistics Reports volume 67, Number 5.

7. OECD 2017 Obesity Update.

8. Health Effects of Overweight and Obesity in 195 Countries Over 25 Years, the GBD Obesity Collaborators; July 6, 2017 N Engl J Med 2017; 377:13-27.

9. Waist circumference and waist-to-height ratio are better predictors of cardiovascular disease risk factors in children

than body mass index, SC Savva et al., Int Nat J Obesity 24, 1453-1458, 2000.

10. National Health and Nutrition Examination Survey 1999-2016 Survey Content Brochure.

Chapter 3: Long-Term Behavioral Change

1. Baumeister, Roy F., and John Tierney. Willpower: Rediscovering the greatest human strength. Penguin; 2011.

2. Mischel Walter, Ozlem Ayduk, Marc G. Berman, B.J. Casey, Ian H. Gotlib, John Jonides, Ethan Kross, Theresa Teslovich, Nicole L. Wilson, Vivian Zayas, and Yuichi Shoda. "'Willpower' over the life span: decomposing self-regulation". Social Cognitive and Affective Neuroscience. 6.2 (2011 Apr.): 252-256.

3. Song HS and Lehrer PH. "The effects of specific respiratory rates on heart rate and heart rate variability". Applied Psychophysiology and Biofeedback. 28.1 (2003 Mar.)

4. Martarelli Danielle Mario Cocchioni, Stefania Scuri, and Pierluigi Pompei. "Diaphragmatic Breathing Reduces Exercise-Induced Oxidative Stress". Evidence Based Complementary and Alternative Medicine; 2011.

5. Oaten M and Cheng K. "Longitudinal gains in self-regulation from regular physical exercise". British Journal of Health Psychology. 11.4 (2006 Nov.): 717-733.

6. Bowen Sarah and Marlatt Alan. "Surfing the urge: Brief mindfulness-based intervention for college student smokers". Psychology of Addictive Behaviors. 23.4 (2009 Dec.): 666-671.

7. Fowler, James H. and Nicholas A. Christakis; 2008. Dynamic spread of happiness in a large social network: longitudinal analysis over 20 years in the Framingham Heart Study. British Medical Journal 337, no. a2338: 1-9.

8. Noël Xavier PhD, Martial Van Der Linden PhD, and Antoine Bechara PhD. "The Neurocognitive Mechanisms of Decision-making, Impulse Control, and Loss of Willpower to Resist Drugs". Psychiatry. 3.5 (2006 May): 30-41.

Chapter 4: How We Get Fat— Sugar Addiction

1. Avena NM, Rada P., Hoebel BG. Evidence for sugar addiction: behavioral and neurochemical effects of intermittent, excessive sugar intake. Neurosci Biobehav Rev. 2007; 32(1): 20-39.

2. Ahmed SH, Guillem K., Vandaele Y. Sugar addiction: pushing the drug-sugar analogy to the limit. Curr Opin Clin Nutr Metab Care. 2013 Jul; 16(4): 434-9.

3. Intense Sweetness Surpasses Cocaine Reward. Magalie Lenoir, Fuschia Serre, Lauriane Cantin, and Serge H. Ahmed.

4. Austin J, Marks D. Hormonal regulators of appetite. Int J Pediatr Endocrinol. 2008; 2009: 141753.

Chapter 5: Age Can Change Your Body

1. Flegal Kathrine M. PhD., Margaret D. Carroll MSPH; Brian K. Kit MD; and Cynthia L. Ogden PhD. "Prevalence of Obesity and Trends in the Distribution of Body Mass Index Among US Adults, 1999-2010". Journal of the American Medical Association. 307.5 (2012 Feb.): 491-497.

2. Erickson Kirk I., Michelle W. Voss, Ruchika Shaurya Prakash, Chandramallika Basake, Amanda Szabo, Laura Chaddock, Jennifer S. Kim, Susie Heob, Heloisa Alves, Siobhan M. White, Thomas R. Wojcickif, Emily Mailey, Victoria J. Vieira, Stephen A. Martin, Brandt D. Pence, Jeffrey A. Woods, Edward McAuley, and Arthur F. Kramer. "Exercise training increases size of hippocampus and improves memory". Proceedings of the National Academy of Sciences of the United States of America. 108.7 (2011 Feb.): 3017-3011.

3. Hartz Arthur J, Mary E. Fischer, Gordon Bril, Sheryl Kelber, David Rupley Jr, Barry Oken, and Alfred A. Rimm. "The association of obesity with joint pain and osteoarthritis in the HANES data". Journal of Chronic Diseases. 39.4 (1986): 311-319.

4. Turano, Kathleen A. PhD; Broman, Aimee T. MS; Bandeen-Roche, Karen PhD; Munoz, Beatriz MS; Rubin, Gary S. PhD; and West, Sheila K. PhD. "Association of Visual Field Loss and Mobility Performance in Older Adults: Salisbury Eye Evaluation Study". Optometry and Vision Science. 81.5 (2004 May): 298-307.

5. Makrantonaki E and Zouboulis CC. "The skin is a mirror of the aging process in the human organism—State of the art and results of the aging research in the German National Genome Research Network 2 (NGFN-2)". Experimental Gerontology. 42.9 (2007 Sept.): 879-886.

6. O'Flaherty Ellen J. "Modeling Normal Aging Bone Loss, with Consideration of Bone Loss in Osteoporosis". Toxicology Sciences. 55.1 (2000): 171-188.

7. Faulkner John A., Lisa M. Larkin, Dennis R. Claflin and Susan V. Brooks. "Age-Related Changes in the Structure and Function of Skeletal Muscles". Clinical and Experimental Pharmacology and Physiology. 34.11 (2007 Nov.): 1091-1096.

8. Waters DL, Baumgartner RN and Garry PJ. "Sarcopenia: current perspectives". The Journal of Nutrition, Health & Aging. 4.3 (2000): 133-139.

9. Mott John W., Jack Wang, John C. Thornton, David B. Allison, Steven B. Heymsfield, and Richard N. Pierson Jr. "Relation between body fat and age in 4 ethnic groups". The American Journal of Clinical Nutrition. 69.5 (1999 May): 107-1013.

10. Wroblewski AP, Amati F., Smiley MA, Goodpaster B., and Wright V. "Chronic exercise preserves lean muscle mass in masters athletes". The Physician and Sportsmedicine. 39.3 (2011): 172-178.

11. Fujita Satoshi and Elena Volpi. "Amino Acids and Muscle Loss with Aging". The Journal of Nutrition. 136.1 (2006 Jan): 277S-280S.

12. Zemuda Joseph M., Paul D. Thompson, and Stephen J. Winters. "Exercise increases serum testosterone and sex hormone—binding globulin levels in older men". Metabolism. 45.8 (1996 Aug.): 935-939.

13. Enns Deborah L., and Peter M. Tildus. "Estrogen influences satellite cell activation and proliferation following downhill running in rats". Journal of Applied Physiology. 104.2 (2008 Feb.): 347-353.

14. NO REFERENCE

15. Shalender Bhasin, M.D.; Thomas W. Storer, Ph.D.; Nancy Berman, Ph.D.; Carlos Callegari, M.D.; Brenda Clevenger, B.A.; Jeffrey Phillips, M.D.; Thomas J. Bunnell, B.A.; Ray Tricker, Ph.D.; Aida Shirazi, R.Ph.; and Richard Casaburi, Ph.D., M.D.N. (July 4, 1996) "The Effects of Supraphysiologic Doses of Testosterone on Muscle Size and Strength in Normal Men."

16. Cangrmi Roberto, Alberto J. Friedmann, John O. Holloszy, and Luigi Fontana. "Long-term effects of calorie restriction on serum sex-hormone concentrations in men". Aging Cell. (2010 Jan): 236-242.

17. Tamiyama Janet A. PhD.; Traci Mann, Ph.D.; Danielle Vinas, B.A.; Jeffrey M. Hunger, B.A.; Jill DeJager, MPH., RD; and Shelley E. Taylor, Ph.D. "Low Calorie Dieting Increases Cortisol". Psychosomatic Medicine. (2010 May): 357-364.

18. Keys, A. Brožek; J. Henschel; A. Mickelsen O.; and Taylor H.L. The Biology of Human Starvation (2 volumes), University of Minnesota Press, 1950.

Chapter 6: Obesity Defined

19. Park Yong-Woo, MD, PhD; Shankuan Zhu, MD, PhD; Latha Palaniappan, MD; Stanley Heshka, PhD; Mercedes R. Carnethon, PhD; and Steven B. Heymsfield, MD. "The Metabolic Syndrome: Prevalence and Associated Risk Factor Findings in the US Population From the Third National Health and Nutrition Examination Survey, 1988-1994". Archives of Internal Medicine. (2003 Feb.): 427-436.

20. Fontaine Kevin R., PhD; David T. Redden, PhD; Chenxi Wang, MD; Andrew O. Westfall, MS; David B. Allison, PhD, et al. "Years of Life Lost Due to Obesity". Journal of the American Medical Association. (2003 Jan.): 187-193.

21. Huxley R., S. Mendis, E. Zheleznyakov, S. Reddy, and J. Chan. "Body mass index, waist circumference and waist-hip ratio as predictors of cardiovascular risk—a review of the literature". European Journal of Clinical Nutrition. (2010): 16-22.

22. Jean-Pierre Després, Body Fat Distribution and Risk of Cardiovascular Disease, 2012—Circulation 1301-1313.

23. Waist circumference and waist-to-height ratio are better predictors of cardiovascular disease risk factors in children than body mass index, SC Savva et al, Int Nat J. 1453-1458, 2000.

24. Mohammed B.S., Cohen S., Reeds D., Young V.L., Klein S. "Long-term effects of large-volume liposuction on metabolic risk factors for coronary heart disease". (2008 Dec): 2648-51.

25. DiGiorgi M., MS, MPH; Daniel J. Rosen, MD; Jenny J. Choi, MD; Luca Milone, MD; Beth Schrope, MD PhD; Lorraine Olivero-Rivera, DNP, FNP-BC; Nancy Restuccia, MS, RD; Sara Yuen, MS; McKenzie Fisk, MS; William B. Inabnet, MD; Marc Bessler, MD. "Re-emergence of diabetes after gastric bypass in patients with mid-to-long-term follow-up". Surgery for Obesity and Related Diseases. (2010 May): 249-253.

26. Golomb Inbal, BSC; Matan Ben David, MD; Adi Glass, BSC; Tamara Kolitz, MD; Andrei Keidar, MD. "Long-term Metabolic Effects of Laparoscopic Sleeve Gastrectomy". Journal of the American Medical Association Surgery. (2015 Nov.): 1051-1057.

27. King W.C., Chen J., Mitchell J.E., Kalarchian M.A., Steffen K.J., Engel S.G., Courcoulas A.P., Pories W.J., Yanovski S.Z. Prevalence of Alcohol Use Disorders Before and After Bariatric Surgery; 2012

Chapter 7: How Your Body Works

1. Manois Yiannis, Vassiliki Costarelli, Maria Kolotourou, Katerina Kondakis, Chara Tzavara and George Moschonis. "Prevalence of obesity in preschool Greek children, in relation to parental characteristics and region of residence". BioMed Central Public Health. (2007 Jul.): 178.

2. Feldman M., B. Cryer, K.E. McArthur, B.A. Huet, E. Lee. "Effects of aging and gastritis on gastric acid and pepsin secretion in humans: A prospective study". Gastroenterology. (1996 Apr.): 1043-1052.

3. Heilbronn L.K., de Jonge L., Frisard M.I., et al. Effect of 6-Month Calorie Restriction on Biomarkers of Longevity, Metabolic Adaptation, and Oxidative Stress in Overweight Individuals: A Randomized Controlled Trial. (2006): 1539–1548.

4. Teicholz, Nina. The big fat surprise: why butter, meat and cheese belong in a healthy diet. Simon and Schuster, 2014.

5. Saturated fat and cardiovascular disease: the discrepancy between the scientific literature and dietary advice; Hoenselaar R1; (2012).

6. Long-term persistence of hormonal adaptations to weight loss. Sumithran P1, Prendergast L.A., Delbridge E., Purcell K., Shulkes A., Kriketos A., Proietto J.; (2011).

7. Mietus-Snyder Michele L. and Robert H. Lustig. "Childhood Obesity: Adrift in the 'Limbic Triangle'" Annual Review of Medicine. (2008 Feb.): 147-162.

8. Guo Shumei S. and William Cameron Chumlea. "Tracking of body mass index in children in relation to overweight in adulthood." American Journal of Physiology. (2007): 145S-148S.

9. Guo Shumei S., Christine Zeller, William Cameron Chumlea, and Roger M. Siervogel. "Aging, body composition, and lifestyle: the Fels Longitudinal Study." American Journal of Clinical Nutrition. (1999): 405-411.

10. Ahima Rexford S. "Connecting obesity, aging and diabetes". Nature Medicine. (2009): 996-997.

11. Tchkonia Tamara, Dean E. Morbeck, Thomas Von Zglinicki, Jan Van Deursen, Joseph Lustgarten, Heidi Scrable, Sundeep Khosla, Michael D. Jensen and James L. Kirkland. "Fat tissue, aging, and cellular senescence". Aging Cell. (2010 Oct.): 667-684.

12. Xu Haiyan, Glenn T. Barnes, Qing Yang, Guo Tan, Daseng Yang, Chieh J. Chou, Jason Sole, Andrew Nichols, Jeffrey S. Ross, Louis A. Tartaglia, and Hong Chen. "Chronic inflammation in fat plays a crucial role in the development of obesity-related insulin resistance". The Journal of Clinical Investigation. (2003 Dec.): 1821-1830.

13. Siri-Tarino Patty W., Qi Sun, Frank B. Hu, and Ronald M. Krauss. "Meta-analysis of prospective cohort studies evaluating the association of saturated fat with cardiovascular disease". The American Journal of Clinical Nutrition. (2010 Jan.): 535-546.

14. Micha Renata and Dariush Mozaffarian. "Saturated Fat and Cardiometabolic Risk Factors, Coronary Heart Disease, Stroke, and Diabetes: a Fresh Look at the Evidence". Lipids. (2010 Mar.): 893-905.

15. Schwab U., Lauritzen L., Tholstrup T., et al. Effect of the amount and type of dietary fat on cardiometabolic risk factors and risk of developing type 2 diabetes, cardiovascular diseases, and cancer: a systematic review. Food & Nutrition Research; (2014).

16. Patty W. Siri-Tarino, Qi Sun, Frank B. Hu, Ronald M. Krauss. Meta-analysis of prospective cohort studies evaluating the association of saturated fat with cardiovascular disease. The American Journal of Clinical Nutrition, Volume 91, Issue 3, 1 March 2010, Pages 535–546.

17. Chowdhury R., Warnakula S., Kunutsor S., Crowe F., Ward H.A., Johnson L., Franco O.H., Butterworth A.S., Forouhi N.G., Thompson S.G., Khaw K.T., Mozaffarian D., Danesh J., Di Angelantonio E. Association of dietary, circulating, and supplement fatty acids with coronary risk: a systematic review and meta-analysis. Ann Intern Med; (2014 Mar.) :398-406.

Chapter 8: Ligands, Insulin Resistance and Metabolic Syndrome

1. H. N. Ginsburg and J. Clin Invest. Insulin resistance and cardiovascular disease; (2000): 453-458.

2. Ginsburg Henry H. "Insulin resistance and cardiovascular disease". The Journal of Clinical Investigation. (2000 Aug.): 453-458.

3. Laakso M., S.V. Edelman, G. Brechtel, and A.D. Baron. "Decreased effect of insulin to stimulate skeletal muscle blood flow in obese man. A novel mechanism for insulin resistance". The Journal of Clinical Investigation. (1990 Jun.): 1844-1852.

4. Ford Earl S. MD, MPH; Wayne H. Giles MD, MSc and William H. Dietz MD, PhD. "Prevalence of the Metabolic Syndrome Among US Adults Findings From the Third National Health and Nutrition Examination Survey". The Journal of the American Medical Association. (2002 Jan.): 356-359.

5. Mayes, PA. "Intermediary metabolism of fructose". The American Journal of Clinical Nutrition. (1993 Nov.): 754S–765S.

6. Kasapis Christos, MD; Paul D. Thompson, MD. "The Effects of Physical Activity on Serum C-Reactive Protein and Inflammatory Markers". Journal of the American College of Cardiology. (2005 May): 1563-1569.

7. Albanes D. "Beta-carotene and lung cancer: a case study". The American Journal of Clinical Nutrition. (1999): 1345s-1350s.

8. AREDS Report No. 8. "A Randomized, Placebo-Controlled Clinical Trial of High-Dose Supplementation With Vitamins C and E, Beta Carotene, and Zinc for Age-Related Macular Degeneration and Vision Loss". The Journal of the American Medical Association Opthalmology. (2001 Oct.): 1417-1436.

9. Dröge Wulf. "Free Radicals in the Physiological Control of Cell Function". Physiological Reviews. (2002 Jan.): 47-95.

10. Summers Scott A. and Don H. Nelson. "A Role for Sphingolipids in Producing the Common Features of Type 2 Diabetes, Metabolic Syndrome X, and Cushing's Syndrome". Diabetes. (2005 Mar.): 591-602.

Chapter 9: Diet

1. Eaton Boyd S., M.D., and Melvin Konner, Ph.D. "Paleolithic Nutrition—A Consideration of Its Nature and Current Implications". The New England Journal of Medicine (1985 Jan.): 283-289.

2. Staffan Lindeberg. "Palaeolithic diet ('stone age' diet)". Scandinavian Journal of Food & Nutrition (2005 Jun.): 75–77.

3. Frank M. Sacks, George A. Bray, Vincent J. Carey, Steven R. Smith, Donna H. Ryan, Stephen D. Anton, Katherine McManus, et al. "Comparison of Weight-Loss Diets with Different Compositions of Fat, Protein, and Carbohydrates." New England Journal of Medicine (2009): 859–873.

4. David A. Sinclair. "Toward a unified theory of caloric restriction and longevity regulation". Mechanisms of Aging and Development (2005 Sept.): 987-1002.

5. Roth G.S., Mattison J.A., Ottinger M.A., Chachich M.E., Lane M.A., and Ingram D.K. "Aging in rhesus monkeys: relevance to human health interventions" (2004 Sept.): 1423-1426.

6. Gredilla Ricardo and Gustavo Batja. "Minireview: The Role of Oxidative Stress in Relation to Caloric Restriction and Longevity". Endocrine Society (2011 Apr.): 3713–3717.

7. Chaouachi Anis, John B. Leiper, Hamdi Chtourou, Abdul Rashid Aziz, and Karim Chamari. "The effects of Ramadan intermittent fasting on athletic performance: Recommendations for the maintenance of physical fitness". Journal of Sports Science (2012 Jun.): 53-73.

8. John M. Freeman, Eric H. Kossoff, Adam L. Hartman. "The Ketogenic Diet: One Decade Later". Pediatrics. (2007 Mar.): 535-543.

9. Paoli Antonio, Bianco Antonino and Grimaldi Keith A. "The Ketogenic Diet and Sport: A Possible Marriage?" (2015 Jul.): 153-162.

10. Sandri M., L. Barberi, A.Y. Bijlsma, B. Blaauw, K.A. Dyar, G. Milan, C. Mammucari, C.G.M. Meskers, G. Pallafacchina, A. Paoli, D. Pion, M. Roceri, V. Romanello, A.L. Serrano, L. Toniolo, L. Larsson, A.B. Maier, P. Muñoz-Cánoves, A. Musarò, M. Pende, C. Reggiani, R. Rizzuto and S. Schiaffino. "Signalling pathways regulating muscle mass in aging skeletal muscle. The role of the IGF1-Akt-mTOR-FoxO pathway" (2013 Jun.): 303-323.

11. Leidy H.J. and Campbell W.W. "The effect of eating frequency on appetite control and food intake: brief synopsis of controlled feeding studies". Journal of Nutrition (2011): 154-157.

12. Mifflin M.D., S.T. St. Jeor, L.A. Hill, B.J. Scott, S.A. Daugherty, and Y.O. Koh. "A new predictive equation for resting energy expenditure in healthy individuals". The American Journal of Clinical Nutrition (1990 Feb.): 241-247.

13. Kevin D. Tipton and Robert R. Wolf. "Protein and amino acids for athletes". Journal of Sports Science (2004): 65-79.

14. Peter W. Lemon, PhD. "Beyond the Zone: Protein Needs of Active Individuals". Journal of the American College of Nutrition (2000): 513S-521S.

15. Raben A., Kiens B., Richter E.A., Rasmussen L.B., Svenstrup B., Micic S., and Bennett P. "Serum sex hormones and endurance performance after a lacto-ovo vegetarian and a mixed diet". Medicine and Science in Sports and Exercise (1992): 1290-1297.

16. Lyne E. Norton, Gabriel J. Wilson, Donald K. Layman, Christopher J. Moulton, and Peter J. Garlick. "Leucine content of dietary proteins is a determinant of postprandial skeletal muscle protein synthesis in adult rats". Nutrition and Metabolism (2012 Jul.): 67.

17. Cara L. Frankenfeld, Charlotte Atkinsona, Wendy K. Thomasa, Alex Gonzaleza, Tuija Jokela, Kristiina Wähäläa, Stephen M. Schwartza, Shuying S. Lia, and Johanna W. Lampe. British Journal of Nutrition (2005 Dec.): 873-876.

18. CDC, NCHS. Underlying Cause of Death 1999-2013 on CDC WONDER Online Database, released 2015. Data is from the Multiple Cause of Death Files, 1999-2013, as compiled from data provided by the 57 vital statistics jurisdictions through the Vital Statistics Cooperative Program. Accessed Feb. 3, 2015.

19. Mozaffarian D., Benjamin E.J., and Go A.S. "Heart Disease and Stroke Statistics—2015 Update". Circulation (2015).

20. Keys Ancel, PhD., F.A.P.H.A. "Prediction and Possible Prevention of Coronary Disease". American Journal of Public Health (1953 Nov): 1399-1407.

21. Chawdhury Rajiv, MD, PhD; Samantha Warnakula, MPhil; Setor Kunutsor, MD, MSt; Francesca Crowe, PhD; Heather A. Ward, PhD; Laura Johnson, PhD; Oscar H. Franco, MD, PhD; Adam S. Butterworth, PhD; Nita G. Forouhi, MRCP, PhD; Simon G. Thompson, FMedSci; Kay-Tee Khaw, FMedSci; Dariush Mozaffarian, MD, DrPH; John Danesh, FRCP; and Emanuele Di Angelantonio, MD, PhD. "Association of Dietary, Circulating, and Supplement Fatty Acids With Coronary Risk: A Systematic Review and Meta-analysis". Annals of Internal Medicine (2014 Mar.): 398-406.

22. Dontas, Anastasios S., Nicholas S. Zerefos, Demosthenes B. Panagiotakos, Cleo Vlachou, and Dimitrios A. Valis. "Mediterranean diet and prevention of coronary heart disease in the elderly (vol 2, pg 109, 2007)." CLINICAL INTERVENTIONS IN AGING 3, no. 2 (2008): 397-397.

23. Willett W.C. "The Mediterranean diet: science and practice". Public Health Nutrition (2006 Feb.): 105-110.

24. Oh Kyungwon, Frank B. Hu, JoAnn E. Manson, Meir J. Stampfer and Walter C. Willett. "Dietary Fat Intake and Risk of Coronary Heart Disease in Women: 20 Years of Follow-up of the Nurses' Health Study". American Journal of Epidemiology (2005): 672-679.

25. Journal of Atherosclerosis Research Cardiovascular disease in the Masai. G.V. Mann, R.D. Shaffer, R.S. Anderson, H.H. Sandstead, H. Prendergast, J.C. Mann, S. Rose, J. Powell-Jackson, S. Moitanik, J. Ol Monah, S.M. Isaac Onesimo, H. Msangi, E. Frank, J. Martin, J. Lane, I. Rasmussen, K. Dicks. Volume 4, Issue 4, 8 July 1964, Pages 289-312.

26. Ho K.J., Biss K., Mikkelson B., Lewis L.A., Taylor C.B. The Masai of East Africa: some unique biological characteristics. Arch Pathol (1971 May): 387-410.

27. Fasting-mimicking diet and markers/risk factors for aging, diabetes, cancer, and cardiovascular disease. Wei M1, Brand-horst S1, Shelehchi M1, Mirzaei H1, Cheng CW1, Budniak J1, Groshen S2, Mack WJ2, Guen E1, Di Biase S1, Cohen P1, Morgan TE1, Dorff T3, Hong K4, Michalsen A5, Laviano A6, Longo VD7, 8. (2017 Feb).

28. Johnston Carol S., Sherrie L. Tjonn, and Pamela D. Swan. "High-Protein, Low-Fat Diets Are Effective for Weight Loss and Favorably Alter Biomarkers in Healthy Adults". American Journal of Clinical Nutrition (2004 Mar.): 1055-1061.

29. Gelfand R.A. and Barrett E.J. "Effect of physiologic hyperin-sulinemia on skeletal muscle protein synthesis and breakdown in man." The Journal of Clinical Investigation (1987 Jul.): 1-6.

30. Lane Amy R., Joseph W. Duke, Anthony C. Hackney. "Influ-ence of dietary carbohydrate intake on the free testosterone: cortisol ratio responses to short-term intensive exercise train-ing". European Journal of Applied Physiology (2010 Apr.): 1125-1131.

31. O'Keefe JH, MD, FACC; Kevin A. Bybee, MD; and Carl J. Lavie, MD, FACC. "Alcohol and cardiovascular health: the razor-sharp double-edged sword". Journal of the American College of Cardiology (2007 Sept.): 1009-1014.

32. Renaud S.C. and De Longeril M. "Wine, alcohol, platelets, and the French paradox for coronary Heart disease". The Lancet (1992 Jun.): 1523-1526.

33. Rimm Eric B., associate professor; Paige Williams, associate professor; Kerry Fosher, research assistant; Michael Criqui, professor; Meir J. Stampfer, professor. "Moderate alcohol intake and lower risk of coronary heart disease: meta-analysis of effects on lipids and haemostatic factors." British Medical Journal (1999 Dec): 1523-1528.

34. Moderate alcohol consumption as risk factor for adverse brain outcomes and cognitive decline: longitudinal cohort study. Topiwala Anya, Allan Charlotte, Cao Y., Willett W.C., Rimm E.B., Stampfer M.J., Giovannucci E.L. Light to moderate intake of alcohol, drinking patterns, and risk of cancer: results from two prospective US cohort studies; 2015.

35. Pepino Yanian M., PhD; Courtney D. Tiemann, MPH, MS, RD; Bruce W. Patterson, PhD; Burton M. Wice, PhD; and Samuel Klein, MD. "Sucralose Affects Glycemic and Hormonal Responses to an Oral Glucose Load". Diabetes Care (2013 Sept.): 2530-2535.

36. "Ingestion of Diet Soda Before a Glucose Load Augments Glucagon-Like Peptide-1 Secretion." Corresponding author: Rebecca J. Brown, brownrebecca@mail.nih.gov.

37. Fredholm Bertil B. "Adenosine, Adenosine Receptors and the Actions of Caffeine". Basic and Clinical Pharmacology and Toxicology (1995 Feb.): 93-101.

38. Dulloo A.G., C.A. Geissler, T. Horton, A. Collins, and D.S.

Miller. "Normal caffeine consumption: influence on thermogenesis and daily energy expenditure in lean and postobese human volunteers." The American Journal of Clinical Nutrition (1989 Jan.): 44-50.

39. Doherty M. and Smith P.M. "Effects of caffeine ingestion on exercise testing: a meta-analysis". International Journal of Sport Nutrition and Exercise Metabolism (2004): 626-646.

40. XingChun Wang, Huan Liu, Jiaqi Chen, Yan Li, and Shen Qu. "Multiple Factors Related to the Secretion of Glucagon-Like Peptide-1." International Journal of Endocrinology, vol. 2015, Article ID 651757, 11 pages, 2015.

41. Mann T1, Tomiyama A.J., Westling E., Lew A.M., Samuels B., Chatman J. Am Psychol (2007 Apr): 220-33; Medicare's search for effective obesity treatments: diets are not the answer.

42. Priya Sumithran, M.B., B.S.; Luke A. Prendergast, Ph.D.; Elizabeth Delbridge, Ph.D.; Katrina Purcell, B.Sc.; Arthur Shulkes, Sc.D.; Adamandia Kriketos, Ph.D.; and Joseph Proietto, M.B., B.S., Ph.D. (October 27, 2011): 1597-1604.

43. Ahima R.S., Antwi D.A. Brain regulation of appetite and satiety. Endocrinology and metabolism clinics of North America (2008): 811-823.

44. Müller M.J., Bosy-Westphal A., and Heymsfield S.B. Is there evidence for a set point that regulates human body weight? Medicine Reports (2010).

45. Ultra-Processed Diets Cause Excess Calorie Intake and Weight Gain. Kevin Hall et al. Cell Metabolism (2019): 67-77.

46. The short-chain fatty acid propionate increases glucagon and FFABP4 production, impairing insulin action in mice and humans. Amir Tirosh et al. Science Translational Medicine (2019).

Chapter 10: Summary of Essential Information About Food

1. Centers for Disease Control and Prevention (2017).

2. Chowdhury R., Warnakula S., Kunutsor S., et al. Ann Intern Med (2014): 398-406.

3. Van Vliet S., Burd N.A., Van Loon L.J. (2015): 1981-91.

4. Dreon D.M., Fernstrom H.A., Campos H., et al. Am J Clin Nutr (1998): 828-36.

5. Siri P.W., Krauss R.M. Curt Atheroscler Rep. (2005): 455-59.

6. Nissen S.E.;Ann Intern Med (2016): 555-559.

7. Astrup A., Dyerberg J., Elwood P., et al. Am J Clin Nutr. (2011): 684-88.

8. Bouvard V., Loomis D., Guyton K.Z., et al. Lancet Oncol. (2015): 1599-1600.

9. Mihrshahi S., Ding D., Gale J., et al. Prev Med. (2017): 1-7.

10. Kaczmarczyk M.M., Miller M.J., Freund G.G. Metabolism (2012): 1058-66.

11. Centers for Disease Control and Prevention. https://www.cdc.gov/nchs/fastats/obesity-overweight.html.

12. Ebbeling C.B., Swain J.F., Feldman H.A., et al. (2012): 2627-34.

13. Bazzano L.A., Hu T., Reynolds K., et al. Ann Intern Med. (2014): 309-18.

14. Tobias D.K., Chen M., Manson J.E., et al. Lancet Diabetes, Endocrinol. (2015): 968-79.

15. Mozaffarian D., Ludwig D.S., JAMA (2015): 2421-22.

16. Sanchez-Muniz F.J. Int J. Vitam Nutr Res. (2006): 230-37.

17. Ramsden C.E., Zamora D., Leelarthaepin B., et al. BMJ (2013).

18. Ramsden C.E., et al. BMJ (2016).

19. St-Onge M.P., Jones P.J., Int J. Obes Relat Metab Disord (2003): 1565-71.

20. Freed D.L.J. BMJ (1999): 1023-4.

21. Sturgeon C., Fasano A. Tissue Barriers (2016).

22. Glickman D., Parker L., Sim L.J., Cook H.D.V., Miller E.A., eds. Accelerating progress in obesity prevention: solving the weight of the nation. Washington, DC: National Academies Press, 2012.

23. Ebbeling C.B., Swain J.F., Feldman H.A., et al. JAMA (2012): 2627-34.

24. Ingestion of Diet Soda Before a Glucose Load Augments Glucagon-Like Peptide-1 Secretion. Rebecca J. Brown, MD; Mary Walter, PHD; and Kristina I. Rother, MD, MHSC Diabetes Care (2009 Dec): 2184–2186.

Chapter 11: Fiber in Your Diet is Amazing

1. N.C. Howarth et al. Dietary Fiber and Weight Regulation. (2001): 129-39.

2. J.L. Slavin. Dietary Fiber and Body Weight. (2005): 411-418.

3. Cherbut et al. Involvement of Small Intestinal Motility in Blood Glucose Response to Dietary Fiber in Man. (1994): 675-685.

4. Short-chain Fatty Acids Stimulate Leptin Production in Adipocytes Through the G Protein-Coupled Receptor GPR41. Yumei Xiong, Norimasa Miyamoto, Kenji Shibata, Mark A. Valasek, Toshiyuki Motoike, Rafal M. Kedzierski, Masashi Yanagisawa. Proceedings of the National Academy of Sciences; Jan. 2004: 1045-1050.

5. A. Psichas, M. Sleeth, K. Murphy, et al. The Short Chain Fatty Acid Propionate Stimulates GLP-1 and PYY Secretion Via Free Fatty Acid Receptor 2 in Rodents. (2015): 424-429.

6. The Fermentable Fibre Inulin Increases Postprandial Serum Short-Chain Fatty Acids and Reduces Free Fatty Acids and Ghrelin in Healthy Subjects. Joshua Tarini, Thomas M.S. Woleve, Joshua Tarini. Applied Physiology, Nutrition, and Metabolism; 2010: 9-16.

7. D.E. King et al. Trends in Dietary Fiber Intake in the United States, 1999-2008.

8. Alyssa N. Crittenden and Stephanie L. Schnorr. Current Views on Hunter-Gatherer Nutrition and the Evolution of the Human Diet. AJPA Yearbook; Nov. 2016.

9. Schley et al. The Immune Enhancing Effects of Dietary Fibers and Prebiotics. British Journal of Nutrition; p221-230.

10. M. Luu, K. Weigand, F. Wedi, et al. Regulation of the Effector Function of CD8+ T-Cells by Gut Microbiota-Derived Metabolite Butyrate; (2018).

Chapter 12: Exercise is the Missing Ingredient

1. Wen Chi Pang, MD, DrPH, Wai J.P., Tsai M.K., Yang Y.C., Cheng T.Y., Lee M.C., Chan H.T., Tsao C.K., Tsai S.P., and Wu X. "Minimum amount of physical activity for reduced mortality and extended life expectancy: a prospective cohort study." Lancet (2011 Oct.): 1244-1253.

2. Rennie K.L., McCarthy N., Yazdgerdi S., Marmot M., and Brunner E. "Association of the metabolic syndrome with both vigorous and moderate physical activity". International Journal of Epidemiology (2003 Aug.): 600-606.

3. Carroll Sean and Mike Dudfield. "What is the Relationship Between Exercise and Metabolic Abnormalities?" Sports Medicine (2004 May): 371-418.

4. Tjønna Arnt Erik, Sang Jun Lee, Øivind Rognmo, Tomas O. Stølen, Anja Bye, Per Magnus Haram, Jan Pål Loennechen, Qusai Y. Al-Share, Eirik Skogvoll, Stig A. Slørdahl, Ole J. Kemi, Sonia M. Najjar, and Ulrik Wisløff. "Aerobic Interval Training Versus Continuous Moderate Exercise as a Treatment for the Metabolic Syndrome". Circulation. (2008 Jul.): 346-354.

5. Holloszy J.O. "Regulation by exercise of skeletal muscle content of mitochondria and GLUT4". Journal of Physiology and Pharmacology. 59 Suppl-7 (2008): 5-18.

6. Elizabeth V. Menshikova, Vladimir B. Ritov, Liane Fairfull, Robert E. Ferrell, David E. Kelley, and Bret H. Goodpaster. "Effects of Exercise on Mitochondrial Content and Function in Aging Human Skeletal Muscle". The Journal of Gerontology Series A (2005 Dec.): 534-540.

7. Thuy S., Ladurner R., Volynets V., Wagner S., Strahl S., Königsrainer A., Maier K.P., Bischoff S.C., and Bergheim I. "Nonalcoholic fatty liver disease in humans is associated

with increased plasma endotoxin and plasminogen activator inhibitor 1 concentrations and with fructose intake". The Journal of Nutrition (2008): 1452-1455.

8. Mark A. Williams, William L. Haskell, Philip A. Ades, Ezra A. Amsterdam, Vera Bittner, Barry A. Franklin, Meg Gulanick, Susan T. Laing and Kerry J. Stewart. "Resistance Exercise in Individuals With and Without Cardiovascular Disease: 2007 Update." Circulation. (2007 Jul.): 572-584.

9. Manias Karen, Debbie McCabe, and Nick Bishop. "Fractures and recurrent fractures in children; varying effects of environmental factors as well as bone size and mass." (2006 Sept.): 652-657.

10. McPherron A.C., Guo T., Bond N.D., Gavrilova O. Increasing muscle mass to improve metabolism. Adipocyte. (2013): 92–98.

Chapter 13: How to be Strong, Robust, and Healthy

1. Al-Mallah M.H., Keteyian S.J., Brawner C.A., Whelton S., and Blaha M.J. "Rationale and design of the Henry Ford Exercise Testing Project (the FIT project)." Clinical Cardiology (2014 Aug.): 456-461.

2. Lee I-Min, MBBS, ScD; Chung-cheng Hsieh, ScD; Ralph S. Paffenbarger Jr., MD, DrPH. "Exercise Intensity and Longevity in Men; The Harvard Alumni Health Study". Journal of the American Medical Association (1995 Apr.): 1179-1184.

3. Michael Kent. Oxford Dictionary of Sports Science and Medicine Vol. 10. Oxford University Press (2006).

4. Safdar A., Little J.P., Stokl A.J., Hettinga B.P., Akhtar M., Tarnopolsky M.A. Exercise increases mitochondrial PGC-1alpha content and promotes nuclear-mitochondrial cross-talk to coordinate mitochondrial biogenesis (2011).

5. Mead GE1, Morley W., Campbell P., Greig C.A., McMurdo M., Lawlor D.A. Cochrane Database Syst Rev. 2008 Oct 8.

6. Izabela Z. Schultz, Robert J. Gatchel. Psychology Clinical practice guidelines no 14. Rockville, MD: Agency for Health Care Policy and Research, US Dept. of Health and Human Services. L. Altchiler & R. Motta (1994). Effects of aerobic and non-aerobic exercise on anxiety, absenteeism and job satisfaction. Journal of Clinical Psychology, 829–840.

7. Abby C. King, Roy F. Oman, Glenn S. Brassington, Donald L. Bliwise, William L. Haskell. Moderate-Intensity Exercise and Self-rated Quality of Sleep in Older Adults: A Randomized Controlled Trial (1997).

8. A Randomized Controlled Trial of the Effect of Exercise on Sleep. Nalin A. Singh, Karen M. Clements, Maria A. Fiatarone. Volume 20, Issue 2, 1 January 1997, Pages 95–101.

9. Sports Medicine, May 1988, Volume 5, Issue 5, pg 303–311. Cite as Heart Rate and Exercise Intensity During Sports Activities.

10. A Recommendation From the Centers for Disease Control and Prevention and the American College of Sports Medicine. Russell R. Pate, PhD; Michael Pratt, MD, MPH; Steven N. Blair, PED; William L. Haskell, PhD; Caroline A. Macera, PhD; Claude Bouchard, PhD; David Buchner, MD, MPH; Walter Ettinger, MD; Gregory W. Heath, DHSc; Abby C. King, PhD; Andrea Kriska, PhD; Arthur S. Leon, MD; Bess H. Marcus, PhD; Jeremy Morris, MD; Ralph S. Paffenbarger Jr., MD; Kevin Patrick, MD; Michael L. Pollock, PhD; James M. Rippe, MD; James Sallis, PhD; Jack H. Wilmore, PhD.

11. Exercise training increases sarcolemmal and mitochondrial fatty acid transport proteins in human skeletal muscle. Jason L. Talanian, Graham P. Holloway, Laelie A. Snook, George J.F. Heigenhauser, Arend Bonen, Lawrence L. Spriet. American Journal of Physiology—Endocrinology and Metabolism; Vol. 299, No. 2 (8 July 2010).

12. Foster C., Farland C.V., Guidotti F., et al. The Effects of High Intensity Interval Training vs. Steady State Training on Aerobic and Anaerobic Capacity. Journal of Sports Science & Medicine (2015): 747-755.

13. Gibala M. "Molecular responses to high-intensity interval exercise." Applied Physiology, Nutrition, and Metabolism (2009 May): 428-432.

14. Billat L. Véronique. "Interval Training for Performance: A Scientific and Empirical Practice." Sports Medicine. (2001 Jan.): 13-31.

15. Gonzalez J.T. et al. "Carbohydrate Availability as a Regulator of Energy Balance With Exercise." Exercise and Sport Science Reviews (2019): 215-222.

Chapter 14: The First Thing to do in the Gym

1. Barnes M.F. (1997).

2. Fowles J.R., D. G. Sale, and J. D. MacDougall. "Reduced strength after passive stretch of the human plantarflexors." Journal of Applied Physiology (2000 Sept.): 1179-1188.

3. Bandy W.D. and Irion J.M. "The effect of time on static stretch on the flexibility of the hamstring muscles." Physical Therapy. (1994 Sept.): 845-850.

4. Kubo Keitaro, Ikebukuro, Toshihiro; Yata, Hideaki; Tsunoda, Naoya; and Kanehisa, Hiroaki. "Time Course of Changes in Muscle and Tendon Properties During Strength Training and Detraining." Journal of Strength and Conditioning Research (2010 Feb.): 322-331.

5. Leitzmann Michael F., MD, DrPH; Yikyung Park, ScD; Aaron Blair, PhD; Rachel Ballard-Barbash, MD; Traci Mouw, MPH; Albert R. Hollenbeck, PhD; and Arthur Schatzkin, MD, DrPH. "Physical Activity Recommendations and Decreased Risk of Mortality." Archive of Internal Medicine (2007 Dec.): 2453-2460.

6. Thompson Paul D., David Buchner, Ileana L. Piña, Gary J. Balady, Mark A. Williams, Bess H. Marcus, Kathy Berra, Steven N. Blair, Fernando Costa, Barry Franklin, Gerald F. Fletcher, Neil F. Gordon, Russell R. Pate, Beatriz L. Rodriguez, Antronette K. Yancey, and Nanette K. Wenger. "Exercise and Physical Activity in the Prevention and Treatment of Atherosclerotic Cardiovascular Disease." Circulation. (2003 Jun.): 3109-3116.

7. Nader, G.A. Concurrent Strength and Endurance Training: From Molecules to Man. Med. Sci. Sports Exerc., Vol. 38, No. 11, pp 1965-1970, 2006.

8. Acute Energy Deprivation Affects Skeletal Muscle Protein Synthesis and Associated Intracellular Signaling Proteins in Physically Active Adults. The Journal of Nutrition, Volume 140, Issue 4, April 2010, Pages 745–751. Stefan M. Pasiakos, Lisa M. Vislocky, et al.

9. Beverly A. Bullen, Sc.D.; Gary S. Skrinar, Ph.D.; Inese Z. Beitins, M.D.; Gretchen von Mering, B.S.; Barry A. Turnbull, M.A.; and Janet W. McArthur, M.D. "Induction of Menstrual Disorders by Strenuous Exercise in Untrained Women." The New England Journal of Medicine (1985 May): 1349-1353.

10. James H. O'Keef, MD; Harshal R. Patil, MD; Carl J. Lavie, MD; Anthony Magalski, MD; Robert A. Vogel, MD; and Peter A. McCullough, MD, MPH. "Potential Adverse Cardiovascular Effects From Excessive Endurance Exercise." Mayo Clinic Proceedings (2012 Jun.): 587-595.

11. Kahanov Leamor, Lindsey E. Eberman, Kenneth E. Games, and Mitch Wasik. "Diagnosis, treatment, and rehabilitation of stress fractures in the lower extremity in runners." Journal of Sports Medicine (2015 Mar.): 87-95.

12. "Myoglobinuria, rhabdomyolysis and marathon running." Q.J. Med, New series XLVII (1978): 463-472.

13. The Effect of Early Whole-Body Vibration Therapy on Neuromuscular Control After Anterior Cruciate Ligament Reconstruction: A Randomized Controlled Trial. Chak Lun Allan Fu, MSc; Shu Hang Patrick Yung, MD; Kan Yip Billy Law, MD; et al. The Am J Sports Med (2013): 804-814.

14. Kimberly S. Peer, Jacob E. Barkley, and Danielle M. Knapp. The Acute Effects of Local Vibration Therapy on Ankle Sprain and Hamstring Strain Injuries. The Physician and Sportsmedicine: 31-38.

15. C. Button, N. Anderson, C. Bradford, et al. The Effect of Multidirectional Mechanical Vibration on Peripheral Circulation of Humans. Clinical Physiology and Functional Imaging (June 6, 2007).

16. Clark M. et al. Editors (2014). NASM Essentials of Personal Fitness Training. Jones and Bartlett Learning 134-141.

Chapter 15: The Holy Grail—How to Lose Fat and Build Muscle at the Same Time

1. Garthe I.G., T. Raastad, P.E. Refsnes, A. Koivisto, J. Sundgot-Borgen. "Effect of Two Different Weight-Loss Rates on Body Composition and Strength and Power-Related Performance in Elite Athletes." International Journal of Sport Nutrition & Exercise Metabolism (2011 Apr.): 97-104.

2. Weigle D.S., Breen P.A., Matthys C.C. "A high-protein diet induces sustained reductions in appetite, ad libitum caloric intake, and body weight despite compensatory changes in diurnal plasma leptin and ghrelin concentrations." American Journal of Clinical Nutrition (2005): 41-48.

3. Burke L.M. et al. J Sports Science: 17-27.

4. Chin-Chance Catherine, Kenneth S. Polonsky, and Dale A. Schoeller. "Twenty-Four-Hour Leptin Levels Respond to Cumulative Short-Term Energy Imbalance and Predict...." Journal of Clinical Endocrinology and Metabolism (2011 Apr.): 2685-2691.

Chapter 16: Dietary Supplements

1. Madison Park; "Half of Americans Use Supplements," CNN (2015 Oct.)

2. Marina Heinon et al., Ravintolisissa paljon humpuukia (2012).

3. Matthew Herper. "The Truly Staggering Cost of Inventing New Drugs." Forbes/Business. (2012 Feb.)

4. Anahad O'Connor, "Herbal Supplements Are Often Not What They Seem." The New York Times (2013 Nov.)

5. J. Hoffman, J. Kang, N.A. Ratamess, M.W. Hoffman, C.P. Tranchina, and A.D. Faigenbaum. "Examination of a pre-exercise, high energy supplement on exercise performance." Journal of the International Society of Sports and Nutrition (2009 Jan.): 6.

6. S.M. Phillips, "Summer Meeting Nutrition Society." Proceedings of the Nutrition Society (2011 Feb.): 100-103.

7. EFSA Journal (2010): 1818.

8. Consumer Reports (2010 Oct.)

9. Ametaj Burim N. Qendrim Zebeli, Fozia Saleem, Nikolaos Psychogios, Michael J. Lewis, Suzanna M. Dunn, Jianguo Xia, and David S. Wishart. "Metabolomics reveals unhealthy alterations in rumen metabolism with increased proportion of cereal grain in the diet of dairy cows." Metabolomics. (2010 Dec.): 583-594.

10. Charles R. Harper, MD and Terry A. Jacobson, MD. "The Fats of Life: The Role of Omega-3 Fatty Acids in the Prevention of Coronary Heart Disease." Archives of Internal Medicine (2001 Oct.): 2185.

11. W.S. Harris, W.E. Connor, D.R. Illingworth, D.W. Rothrock, and D.M. Foster. "Effects of fish oil on VLDL triglyceride kinetics in humans." Journal of Lipid Research (1990 Sept.): 1549-1558.

12. An Pan, Danxia Yu, Wendy Demark-Wahnefried, Oscar H. Franco, Xu Lin. Meta-analysis of the effects of flaxseed interventions on blood lipids. The American Journal of Clinical Nutrition, Volume 90, Issue 2, August 2009, Pages 288–297.

13. Theodore M. Brasky, Amy K. Darke, Xiaoling Song, Catherine

M. Tangen, Phyllis J. Goodman, Ian M. Thompson, Frank L. Meyskens Jr., Gary E. Goodman, Lori M. Minasian, Howard L. Parnes, Eric A. Klein, and Alan R. Kristal. "Plasma Phospholipid Fatty Acids and Prostate Cancer Risk in the SELECT Trial." Journal of the National Cancer Institute (2013 Jul.): 1132-1141.

14. M.C. Roncaglioni. "N–3 Fatty Acids in Patients with Multiple Cardiovascular Risk Factors." The New England Journal of Medicine (2013 May): 1800-1808.

15. A. Heikkinen, A. Alaranta, I. Helenius, and T. Vasankari. "Dietary supplementation habits and perceptions of supplement use among elite Finnish athletes." International Journal of Sports Nutrition and Exercise Metabolism (2011 Aug.): 271-9.

16. J.L. Sanchez-Benito, E. Sánchez-Soriano, and J. Ginart Suárez. "Unbalanced intake of fats and minerals associated with risk hypertension by young cyclists." Nutrition Hospitalaria. (2007): 552-559.

17. R. Cooper, F. Naclerio, J. Allgrove, and A. Jimenez. Creatine supplementation with specific view to exercise/sports performance: an update. Journal of the International Society of Sports Nutrition (2012).

18. W.J. Kraemer, J.S. Volek, K.L. Clark, S.E. Gordon, S.M. Puhl, L.P. Koziris, J.M. McBride, N.T. Triplett-McBride, M. Putukian, R.U. Newton, K. Hakkinen, J.A. Bush, W.J. Sebastianelli. Influence of exercise training on physiological and performance changes with weight loss in men. Med. Sci. Sports Exerc. (1999): 1320–1329.

19. Strategic creatine supplementation and resistance training in healthy older adults. Darren G. Candow, Emelie Vogt, Sarah Johannsmeyer, Scott C. Forbes, Jonathan P. Farthing. Faculty of Kinesiology & Health Studies, University of Regina.

20. Yen S.S.C., A.J. Morales, and O. Khorram. "Replacement of DHEA in Aging Men and Women Potential Remedial Effects." Annals of the New York Academy of Sciences (1995 Dec.): 128-142.

21. C. Gordon, E. Grace, S.J. Emans, E. Goodman, M.H. Crawford, M.S. Leboff. Changes in bone turnover markers and menstrual function after short-term oral DHEA in young women with anorexia nervosa. J. Bone Miner Res. (1999): 136-145.

22. O.M. Wolkowitz, V.I. Reus, A. Keebler, N. Nelson, M. Friedland, L. Brizendine, E. Roberts. Double-blind treatment of major depression with dehydroepiandrosterone. Am. J. Psychiatry (1999): 646-649.

23. Effects of Testosterone Treatment in Older Men. Peter J. Snyder, M.D., et al; Testosterone Trials Investigators. N. Engl. J. Med. (2016 Feb.): 611-624.

24. Rebecca Vigan, MD, MSCS; Colin I. O'Donnell, MS; Anna E. Barón, PhD; Gary K. Grunwald, PhD; Thomas M. Maddox, MD, MSc; Steven M. Bradley, MD, MPH; Al Barqawi, MD; Glenn Woning, MD; Margaret E. Wierman, MD; Mary E. Plomondon, PhD; John S. Vigan, et al. JAMA (2013): 1829-1836.

25. Normalization of testosterone level is associated with reduced incidence of myocardial infarction and mortality in men. Rishi Sharma, Olurinde A. Oni, Kamal Gupta, Guoqing Chen, Mukut Sharma, Buddhadeb Dawn, Ram Sharma, Deepak Parashara, Virginia J. Savin, John A. Ambrose. European Heart Journal, Volume 36, Issue 40, 21 October 2015, Pages 2706–2715.

26. Rumsfeld, MD, PhD and P. Michael Ho, MD, PhD. "Association of Testosterone Therapy With Mortality, Myocardial Infarction, and Stroke in Men With Low Testosterone Levels." Journal of the American Medical Association (2013 Nov.): 1829-1836. (pg.126)

27. M.R. Stein, R.E. Julis, C.C. Peck, W. Hinshaw, J.E. Sawicki, and J.J. Deller Jr. "Ineffectiveness of human chorionic gonadotropin in weight reduction: a double-blind study." The American Journal of Clinical Nutrition (1976 Sept.): 940-948.

28. Matthew D. Vukovich, Nancy B. Stubbs, and Ruth M. Bohlken. "Body Composition in 70-Year-Old Adults Responds to Dietary β-Hydroxy-β-Methylbutyrate Similarly to That of Young Adults." The Journal of Nutrition (2001 Jul.): 2049-2052.

29. Steven L. Nissen and Rick L. Sharp. "Effect of dietary supplements on lean mass and strength gains with resistance exercise: a meta-analysis." Journal of Applied Physiology (2003 Feb.): 651-659.

30. Prevalence and correlates of vitamin D deficiency in US adults.

31. M.F. Holick. Vitamin D deficiency. N. Engl. J. Med. (2007): 266-81.

32. S. Pilz, W. Marz, B. Wellnitz, et al. Association of vitamin D deficiency with heart failure and sudden cardiac death in a large cross-sectional study of patients referred for coronary angiography. J. Clin. Endocrinol Metab. (2008): 3927-35.

33. M. Hewison. An update on vitamin D and human immunity. Clin. Endocrinol. (2012): 315–325.

34. St. Onge Marie-Pierre and Peter J.H. Jones. "Physiological Effects of Medium-Chain Triglycerides: Potential Agents in the Prevention of Obesity." The Journal of Nutrition (2002 Mar.): 329-332.

35. Branched-chain amino acids and muscle protein synthesis in humans: myth or reality? Robert R. Wolfe. Journal of the International Society of Sports Nutrition (2017).

36. Sarah R. Jackman, Oliver C. Witard, Andrew Philp, Gareth A. Wallis, Keith Baar, Kevin D. Tipton. Branched-Chain Amino

Acid Ingestion Stimulates Muscle Myofibrillar Protein Synthesis following Resistance Exercise in Humans. Frontiers in Physiology (2017).

37. James M. Smoglia, Joseph A. Baur, and Heather A. Hausenblas. "Resveratrol and Health—A Comprehensive Review of Human Clinical Trials." Molecular Nutrition and Food Research (2011 Aug.): 1129-1141.

38. The Therapeutic Potential of Resveratrol: A Review of Clinical Trials. Adi Y. Berman, Rachel A. Motechin, Maia Y. Wiesenfeld, and Marina K. Holz. Precision Oncology 1, Article number 35 (2017).

39. Julia R. Barrett. "The Science of Soy: What Do We Really Know?" Environmental Health Perspectives (2006 Jun.): 352-358.

40. Lu Z.L.; Collaborative Group for China Coronary Secondary Prevention Using Xuezhikang (February 2005).

41. A. Kumar, H. Kaur, P. Devi, et al. Role of coenzyme Q10 (CoQ10) in cardiac disease, hypertension and Meniere-like syndrome. Pharmacology & Therapeutics (2009): 259–268.

42. Bertil B. Fredhom; "Adenosine, Adenosine Receptors and the Actions of Caffeine." Basic and Clinical Pharmacology and Toxicology (1995 Feb.): 93-101.

43. A.G. Dulloo, C.A. Geissler, T. Horton, A. Collins, and D.S. Miller. "Normal caffeine consumption: influence on thermogenesis and daily energy expenditure in lean and postobese human volunteers." The American Journal of Clinical Nutrition (1989): 44-50.

44. M. Doherty and P.M. Smith. "Effects of caffeine ingestion on exercise testing: a meta-analysis." International Journal of Sport Nutrition and Exercise Metabolism (2004 Dec.): 626-646.

45. Reid G. "The scientific basis for probiotic strains of Lacto-bacillus." Applied Environmental Microbiology (1999 Sept.): 3763-3766.

46. Verna EC and Lucak S. "Use of probiotics in gastrointestinal disorders: what to recommend?" Therapeutic Advantages of Gastroenterology (2010 Sept.): 307-319.

47. D.L. Costill, G.P. Dalsky, and W.J. Fink. "Effects of caffeine ingestion on metabolism and exercise performance." Medicine and Science in Sports (1978 Fall): 155-158.

48. A.C. Munhall and S.W. Johnson. "Dopamine-mediated actions of ephedrine in the rat substantia nigra." Brain Research. (2006 Jan.): 96-103.

49. P.G. Shekelle, M.L. Hardy, S.C. Morton, M. Maglione, W.A. Mojica, M.J. Suttorp, S.L. Rhodes, L. Jungvig and J. Gagné. "Efficacy and safety of ephedra and ephedrine for weight loss and athletic performance: a meta-analysis." Journal of the American Medical Association (2003 Mar.): 1537-1545.

50. F. Magkos and S.A. Kavouras. "Caffeine and ephedrine: physiological, metabolic and performance-enhancing effects." Sports Medicine New Zealand (2004): 871-889.

51. A.G. Dulloo, C. Duret, D. Rohrer, L. Girardier, N. Mensi, M. Fathi, P. Chantre, and J. Vandermander. "Efficacy of a green tea extract rich in catechin polyphenols and caffeine in increasing 24-hr energy expenditure and fat oxidation in humans." American Journal of Clinical Nutrition (1999 Dec.): 1040-1045.

52. Martinez Munoz I.Y., Camarillo Romero E.D.S., Garduno Garcia J.J. "Irisin, a Novel Metabolic Biomarker: Present Knowledge and Future Directions." Int J Endocrinol (2018).

Chapter 17: Estrogen Replacement

1. Risks and Benefits of Estrogen Plus Progestin in Healthy Postmenopausal Women; Principal Results From the Women's Health Initiative Randomized Controlled Trial. Writing Group for the Women's Health Initiative Investigators.

2. R.D. Langer. The evidence base for HRT: what can we believe? Climacteric, (2017).

3. Obstetrics and Gynecology International, Volume 2015. A Reappraisal of Women's Health Initiative Estrogen-Alone Trial: Long-Term Outcomes in Women 50–59 Years of Age. Eric Roehm.

4. Vascular Effects of Early Versus Late Postmenopausal Treatment With Estradiol. Howard N. Hodis, M.D.; Wendy J. Mack, Ph.D.; Victor W. Henderson, M.D.; Donna Shoupe, M.D.; Matthew J. Budoff, M.D.; Juliana Hwang-Levine, Pharm.D.; Yanjie Li, M.D.; Mei Feng, M.D.; Laurie Dustin, M.S.; Naoko Kono, M.P.H.; Frank Z. Stanczyk, Ph.D.; Robert H. Selzer, M.S.; and Stanley P. Azen, Ph.D. (2016).

5. Mortality in a cohort of long-term users of hormone replacement therapy: an updated analysis. BJOG: An International Journal of Obstetrics & Gynaecology, Volume 97, Issue 12, Pages 1080-1086, December 1990. Kate Hunt, Martin Vessey, and Klim McPherson.

6. Subclinical cardiovascular disease in postmenopausal women with low/medium cardiovascular risk by the Framingham risk score (2015 Jun).

Chapter 18: Women are Complicated— Hormone Replacement Therapy

1. J.P. Del Río, M.I. Alliende, N. Molina, F.G. Serrano, S. Molina, and P. Vigil. Steroid Hormones and Their Action in Women's Brains: The Importance of Hormonal Balance. Front Public Health (2018): 141.

2. W. Wharton, C.E. Gleason, S.R. Olson, C.M. Carlsson, and S. Asthana. Neurobiological Underpinnings of the Estrogen-Mood Relationship.

3. Hormone Replacement Therapy and Incidence of Acute Myocardial Infarction. Cristina Varas-Lorenzo, Luis A. García-Rodríguez, Susanne Perez-Gutthann, et al.

4. B.D. Pardhe, S. Ghimire, J. Shakya, et al. Elevated Cardiovascular Risks Among Postmenopausal Women: A Community-Based Case Control Study from Nepal.

5. M.E. Mendelsohn and R.H. Karas. The Protective Effects of Estrogen on the Cardiovascular System. The New England Journal of Medicine; (1999 Jun.): 1801-1811.

6. K. Miyagawa, J. Rösch, F. Stanczyk, et al. Medroxyprogesterone Interferes With Ovarian Steroid Protection Against Coronary Vasospasm.

7. R.T. Chlebowski and G.L. Anderson. Changing Concepts: Menopausal Hormone Therapy and Breast Cancer.

8. P. Stute, L. Wildt, and J. Neulen. The Impact of Micronized Progesterone on Breast Cancer Risk: a Systematic Review.

9. D.E.L. Promislow. Senescence in Natural Populations of Mammals: a Comparative Study.

10. S. Zárate, T. Stevnsner, and R. Gredilla. Role of Estrogen and

Other Sex Hormones in Brain Aging. Neuroprotection and DNA Repair.

11. D. Dumitriu, P.R. Rapp, B.S. McEwen, and J.H. Morrison. Estrogen and the Aging Brain: an Elixir for the Weary Cortical Network.

12. The Role of Progesterone and Gaba in PMS/PMDD. Torbjörn Bäckström, Lotta Andréen, Inger Björn, Inga-Maj Johansson, and Magnus Löfgren.

Chapter 19: The Medical Management of Obesity

1. U.S. National Center for Health Statistics, Prevalence of overweight and obesity among adults. Hyattsville, MD: U.S. Department of Health and Human Services, Public Health Service, Centers for Disease Control and Prevention.

2. J.E. Manson, W.C. Willett, M.J. Stampfer, G.A. Colditz, D.J. Hunter, S.E. Hankinson, C.H. Hennekens, and F.E. Speizer. "Body Weight and Mortality Among Women." The New England Journal of Medicine (1995 Sept.): 677-685.

3. World Health Organization. "Obesity: Preventing and Managing the Global Epidemic. Report of a WHO Consultation. Geneva: World Health Organization; 2000." WHO technical report series.

4. R. Abel, M. Modan, D.S. Silverberg, H.E. Eliahou, and B. Modan. "Effect of weight loss without salt restriction on the reduction of blood pressure in overweight hypertensive patients." The New England Journal of Medicine (1978 Jan.): 1-6.

5. P.D. Wood, M.L. Stefanick, D.M. Dreon, B. Frey-Hewitt, S.C. Garay, P.T. Williams, H.R. Superko, S.P. Fortmann, J.J. Albers, K.M. Vranizan, et al. "Changes in plasma lipids and lipoproteins in overweight men during weight loss through dieting as compared with exercise." The New England Journal of Medicine (1988 Nov.)

6. F. Xavier Pi-Sunyer et al. "Clinical guidelines on the identification, evaluation, and treatment of overweight and obesity in adults." American Journal of Clinical Nutrition (1998): 899-917.

7. John A. Orzano, MD, MPH and John G. Scott, MD, PhD. "Diagnosis and Treatment of Obesity in Adults: An Applied Evidence-Based Review." Journal of the American Board of Family Medicine (2004 Sept.): 359-369.

8. Martha L. Skender, MPH, RD; G. Ken Goodrick, PhD; Deborah J. Del Junco, PhD; Rebecca S. Reeves, DrPH, RD; Linda Darnell, PhD; Antonio M. Gotto Jr., MD, and John P. Foreyt, PhD. "Comparison of 2-Year Weight Loss Trends in Behavioral Treatments of Obesity: Diet, Exercise, and Combination Interventions." Journal of the American Dietic Association (1996 Apr.): 342-346.

9. C.K. Haddock, W.S. Poston, P.L. Dill, J.P. Foreyt, and M. Ericsson. "Pharmacotherapy for obesity: a quantitative analysis of four decades of published randomized clinical trials." International Journal of Obesity and Related Metabolic Disorders (2002): 262-273.

10. C. Cercato, V.A. Roizenblatt, C.C. Leança, A. Segal, A.P. Lopes Filho, M.C. Mancini, and A. Halpern. "A randomized double-blind placebo-controlled study of the long-term efficacy and safety of diethylpropion in the treatment of obese subjects." Internal Journal of Obesity (London) (2009 Aug.): 857-865.

11. J.H. Shin and K.M. Gadde. "Clinical utility of phentermine/topiramate (Qsymia™) combination for the treatment of obesity." Diabetes, Metab Syndrome and Obesity: targets and therapy (2013 Apr.): 131-139.

12. S. Woloshin and L.M. Schwartz. "The new weight-loss drugs, lorcaserin and phentermine-topiramate: slim pickings?" Journal of the American Medical Association, Internal Medicine (2014 Apr.): 615-619.

13. J.B. Hauptman, F.S. Jeunet, and D. Hartmann. "Initial studies in humans with the novel gastrointestinal lipase inhibitor Ro 18-0647 (tetrahydrolipstatin)." The American Journal of Clinical Nutrition (1992 Jan.): 309S-313S.

14. S.B. Heymsfield, D.B. Allison, J.R. Vasselli, A. Pietrobelli, D. Greenfeild, and C. Nunez. "Garcinia cambogia (hydroxycitric acid) as a potential antiobesity agent: a randomized controlled trial." The Journal of the American Medical Association (1998 Nov.): 1596-1600.

15. S.Z. Yanovski and J.A. Yanovski. "Long-term drug treatment for obesity: a systematic and clinical review." The Journal of the American Medical Association (2014 Jan.): 74-86.

Chapter 20: In Theory, a Set Point Controls Your Body Weight

1. M.J. Müller, A. Bosy-Westphal, S.B. Heymsfield. "Is there evidence for a set point that regulates human body weight?" F1000 Medicine Reports (2010).

2. "Adaptive reduction in basal metabolic rate in response to food deprivation in humans: a role for feedback signals from fat stores." A.G. Dulloo and J. Jacquet.

3. Long-term persistence of hormonal adaptations to weight loss. P. Sumithran, L.A. Prendergast, E. Delbridge, K. Purcell, A. Shulkes, A. Kriketos, J. Proietto.

4. Reversible biological adaptations in obesity. Per Södersten et al. The Lancet Diabetes & Endocrinology, Volume 3, Issue 5, 314.

5. A. Keys, J. Brožek, A. Henschel, O. Mickelsen, and H.L. Taylor. The Biology of Human Starvation (2 volumes), University of Minnesota Press, 1950.

6. S. Blüher, C.S. Mantzoros. Leptin in Humans: Lessons From Translational Research (2009).

7. The Contribution of Genetics and Environment to Obesity. David Albuquerque, Clévio Nóbrega, Licínio Manco, Cristina Padez. British Medical Bulletin, Volume 123, Issue 1, September 2017, Pages 159–173.

8. Maternal obesity and pregnancy outcome: a study of 287,213 pregnancies in London. N.J. Sebire, M. Jolly, J.P. Harris, J. Wadsworth, M. Joffe, R.W. Beard, and L. Regan. International Journal of Obesity 25 (2001).

9. J.G. Kral, S. Biron, S. Simard, et al. Large maternal weight

loss from obesity surgery prevents transmission of obesity to children who were followed for 2 to 18 years (2006).

10. Successful weight loss maintenance includes long-term increased meal responses of GLP-1 and PYY3-36. Eva Pers, Winning Iepsen, Julie R. Lundgren, Jens Juul Holst, Sten Madsbad, Signe Sørensen Torekov. European Journal of Endocrinology (2016).

Chapter 21: The Optimum Body Unification Theory

1. D.D. Sarbassov, S.M. Ali, and D.M. Sabatini, "Growing roles for the mTOR pathway." Current Opinion in Cell Biology, vol. 17, no. 6, pp. 596–603, 2005.

2. F. Tremblay and A. Marette, "Amino acid and insulin signaling via the mTOR/p70 S6 kinase pathway: a negative feedback mechanism leading to insulin resistance in skeletal muscle cells." The Journal of Biological Chemistry, vol. 276, no. 41, pp. 38052–38060, 2001.

3. Resistance Exercise Initiates mTOR localization in human skeletal muscle; Zhe Song, Daniel R. Moore, et al; Scientific Reports 7, 5028; 2017.

Chapter 22: Human Immunity— Everything You Do

1. C.M. Weyand and J.J. Goronzy. Aging of the Immune System. Mechanisms and Therapeutic Targets.

2. D.B. Palmer. The Effect of Age on Thymic Function.

3. A. Aw and D.B. Palmer. The Origin and Implication of Thymic Involution.

4. C.E. Childs, P.C. Calder, E.A. Miles. Diet and Immune Function.

5. De Heredia et al. Obesity, Inflammation and the Immune System. Proceedings of the Nutrition Society.

6. E.G. Aguilar and W.J. Murphy. Obesity-Induced T-Cell Dysfunction and Implications for Cancer Immunotherapy.

7. J.P. Campbell and J.E. Turner. Debunking the Myth of Exercise-Induced Immune Suppression: Redefining the Impact of Exercise on Immunological Health Across the Lifespan.

8. A.L. de Araujo, L.C. Silva, J.R. Fernandes, Mde S. Matias, L.S. Boas, C.M. Machado, et al. Elderly Men With Moderate and Intense Training Lifestyle Present Sustained Higher Antibody Responses to Influenza Vaccine.

9. J. Wu, L. Zhou, J. Liu, et al. The Efficacy of Thymosin Alpha 1 for Severe Sepsis (ETASS): a Multicenter, Single-Blind, Randomized and Controlled Trial.

10. C.W. Tuthill and R.S. King. Thymosin Alpha 1—a Peptide Immune Modulator With a Broad Range of Clinical Applications.

Chapter 23: Evolution, Progress, Change

1. Tim D. White, Berhane Asfaw, David DeGusta, Henry Gilbert, Gary D. Richards, Gen Suwa, and F. Clark Howell. "Pleistocene Homo sapiens from Middle Awash, Ethiopia," (2003 Apr.): 742-747.

2. Travis Rayne Pickering and Henry T. Bunn. "The Endurance Running Hypothesis, and Hunting and Scavenging in Savanna-Woodlands." Journal of Human Evolution (2007): 434-438.

3. Anthony J. Vita et al. "Aging, Health Risks, and Cumulative Disability." New England Journal of Medicine (1998): 1035-1041.

4. Ricki J. Colman et al. "Caloric restriction reduces age-related and all-cause mortality in rhesus monkeys." Nature communications 5 (2014).

5. A. Keys, J. Brozek, A. Henschel, D. Michelson, and H.L. Taylor. "The Biology of Human Starvation." Minneapolis: University of Minneapolis Press, Vol. 2.

6. De Magalhães, João Pedro, et al. "Genome-environment interactions that modulate aging: powerful targets for drug discovery." Pharmacological Review (2012): 88-101.

7. Bocquet-Appel and Jean-Pierre. "When the World's Population Took Off: The Springboard of the Neolithic Demographic Transition," (2011): 560-561.

8. Oscar H. Franco, Anna Peeters, Luc Bonneux, and Chris de Laet. "Blood Pressure in Adulthood and Life Expectancy With Cardiovascular Disease in Men and Women," (2005 Jun.): 280-286.

9. P. Carrera-Batos et al. Research Reports in Clinical Cardiology, (2011): 15-35.

10. Eric Schlosser, Fast Food Nation: The Dark Side of the All-American Meal, p.35, Houghton Mifflin Harcourt, Kindle edition, (2012).

Chapter 24: Plant-Based Diet?

1. M.J. Orlich, P.N. Singh, J. Sabaté, K. Jaceldo-Siegl, J. Fan, S. Knutsen, and G.E. Fraser. Vegetarian Dietary Patterns and Mortality in Adventist Health Study (2013). JAMA Internal Medicine: 1230–1238.

2. Association of Dietary, Circulating, and Supplement Fatty Acids With Coronary Risk: a Systematic Review and Meta-Analysis. R. Chowdhury, S. Warnakula, S. Kunutsor, F. Crowe, H.A. Ward, L. Johnson, O.H. Franco, A.S. Butterworth, N.G. Forouhi, S.G. Thompson, K.T. Khaw, D. Mozaffarian, J. Danesh, and E. Di Angelantonio.

3. "Calorie Restriction and Aging: Review of the Literature and Implications for Studies in Humans." Leonie K. Heilbronn and Eric Ravussin.

Chapter 25: Telomeres And Longevity

1. A. Ahmid, J. Am. Geriatric. Soc.

2. O.T. Njajou et al. PNAS.

3. O.T. Njajou et al. J. Gerontology; 2009; 860-864.

4. T.J. LaRocca et al. Mech Aging Develop; 2010; 165-167.

5. A.T. Ludlow et al. Med. Sci. Sports Exerc.; 2008; 1764-1771.

6. Beckman and Ames; Physiological Reviews Vol. 78, No. 2, April 1998. The Free Radical Theory of Aging Matures.

7. "A DNA Damage Checkpoint Response in Telomere-Initiated Senescence." d'Adda di Fagagna, P.M. Reaper, L. Clay-Farrace, H. Fiegler, P. Carr, T. Von Zglinicki, G. Saretzki, N.P. Carter, S.P. Jackson.

8. "Cellular Senescence and Tissue Aging in Vivo," P.J. Hornsby.

9. "Identification of a Specific Telomere Terminal Transferase Activity in Tetrahymena Extracts," C.W. Greider and E.H. Blackburn.

10. "Telomerase and the Aging Process," Peter J. Hornsby.

11. B.G. Childs, M. Durik, D.J. Baker, and J.M. van Deursen. "Cellular Senescence in Aging and Age-Related Disease: From Mechanisms to Therapy."

12. "The Role of Senescent Cells in Aging," Jan M. van Deursen (2016): 439-446.

13. D.G. Burton and V. Krizhanovsky. "Physiological and Pathological Consequences of Cellular Senescence," (2014): 4373–4386.

14. "Exercise Prevents Diet-Induced Cellular Senescence in Adipose Tissue." Marissa J. Schafer et al. (2016): 1606-1615.

Chapter 26: Anti-Aging

1. Danielle M. Townsley et al., "Danazol Treatment for Telomere Diseases." New England Journal of Medicine; May 19, 2016.

2. Rodrigo T. Calado et al., "Sex Hormones, Acting on the TERT Gene, Increase Telomerase Activity in Human Primary Hematopoietic Cells."

3. Duk-Chul Lee et al. "Effect of Long-Term Hormone Therapy on Telomere Length in Postmenopausal Women." Yonsei Medical Journal, Vol. 46 (2005).

4. A.M. Valdes, Andrew T., J.P. Gardner, et al. "Obesity, Cigarette Smoking, and Telomere Length in women." Lancet (2005): 662–664

5. S. Pavanello, A.C. Pesatori, L. Dioni, et al. "Shorter Telomere Length in Peripheral Blood Lymphocytes of Workers Exposed to Polycyclic Aromatic Hydrocarbons." Carcinogenesis (2010): 216–221.

6. E.S. Epel, E.H. Blackburn, J. Lin, et al. "Accelerated Telomere Shortening in Response to Life Stress.

7. C. Werner, T. Fürster, T. Widmann, et al. "Physical Exercise Prevents Cellular Senescence in Circulating Leukocytes and in the Vessel Wall."

8. Research Society on Alcoholism (June 26, 2017).

9. A.M. Fretts, B.V. Howard, D.S. Siscovick, L.G. Best, S.A. Beresford, M. Mete, et al. "Processed Meat, but not Unprocessed Red Meat, is Inversely Associated With Leukocyte Telomere Length in the Strong Heart Family Study."

10. J.B. Richards, A.M. Valdes, J.P. Gardner, et al. "Higher serum vitamin D concentrations are associated with longer leukocyte telomere length in women."

11. E. Coluzzi, M. Colamartino, R. Cozzi, et al. "Oxidative stress induces persistent telomeric DNA damage responsible for nuclear morphology change in mammalian cells."

12. A. Rahal, A. Kumar, V. Singh, et al. "Oxidative Stress, Pro-Oxidants, and Antioxidants: the Interplay."

13. N. Barzilai, J.P. Crandall, S.B. Kritchevsky, M.A. Espeland. "Metformin as a Tool to Target Aging."

14. S. Imai and L. Guarente. "It Takes Two to Tango: NAD+ and Sirtuins in Aging/Longevity Control."

15. https://nccih.nih.gov/health/antioxidants/introduction.htm

16. Nadima Shegem, Abeer Nasir, Abdel-Kareem Jbour, Anwar Batieha, Mohammed El-Khateeb, and Kamel Ajlouni. "Effects of Short-Term Metformin Administration on Androgens in Normal Men." Saudi Medical Journal (2002).

17. "Biology of Healthy Aging and Longevity," J.J. Carmona and S. Michan.

Chapter 27: Peptide Therapy

1. D. Rudman, A.G. Feller, H.S. Nagraj, et al. "Effects of Human Growth Hormone in Men Over 60 Years Old."

2. R.F. Walker; "Sermorelin: a Better Approach to Management of Adult-Onset Growth Hormone Insufficiency?" Clinical Interventions in Aging (2006): 307-308.

3. Giovanni Vitale, Giuseppe Pellegrino, Maria Vollery, and Leo J. Hofland. "Role of IGF-1 System in the Modulation of Longevity: Controversies and New Insights From a Centenarian's Perspective." Front Endocrinol (Lausanne) (2019).

INDEX

A

Campbell, Thomas 236
Canada
  Regina, Saskatchewan 178
Carbohydrate cycling 168, 169
Carbohydrates 44, 51, 61, 79, 83, 89, 90, 281
  Healthy 89
  High-glycemic 84, 93, 232
  Intermediate glycemic 166, 168, 255
  Unhealthy 89
Carcinogens 244
Cardiovascular disease 3, 5, 6, 7, 36, 47, 56, 91, 98, 110, 152, 171, 184, 231,
        237, 270, 276, 277, 278, 279, 284, 303
Cardiovascular exercise 110, 118, 119, 134, 153, 171, 216, 256
Cardiovascular interval training 110
CART 19
Casein 175
Casein protein 85
Catechins 192
CCK 19
Celiac disease 102
Centers for Disease Control and Prevention 2, 35, 86, 119, 134, 287, 292, 305
Chiropractic 156
Cholesterol 3, 46, 55, 56, 64, 66, 86, 87, 88, 98, 101, 188, 189, 194, 227, 235, 236
Chylomicrons 64, 185
Cirrhosis 91
Clinton, Bill 235
Coca-Cola 61, 233
Cochrane 117, 292
Coenzyme Q10 68, 189
College of Sports Medicine (ACSM), 159
Colon cancer 99, 100, 184
Comorbidities 202
Consumer Reports 235, 297
Contrave 207
CoQ10 167, 189, 301
Core Exercise 132, 133
Coronary artery disease 2, 6, 16, 40, 54, 55, 56, 59, 63, 66, 73, 86, 87, 88, 90, 91,
        92, 97, 100, 152, 188, 189, 194, 197, 201, 202, 221, 231
Coronary atherosclerosis 193
Coronary heart disease 55, 86, 88, 91, 101, 170, 237, 276, 283, 285
Cortisol 8, 33, 50, 51, 52, 64, 80, 90, 103, 110, 116, 284
C-reactive protein 5, 56, 63, 66, 91, 221, 256
Creatine 178, 298
Crestor 194

Cyrus, Miley 235
Cytokines 54, 214, 220, 241, 247
Cytoskeleton 214

D

Danazol 243
Decline in sex hormone levels 28, 198
Decreased activity 27
Degenerative joint disease 25, 53, 201
DeGeneres, Ellen 235
Dementia 2, 16, 54, 91, 97, 198, 221
Depression 93, 117, 152, 181, 190, 197, 200, 206, 207, 228, 299
DEXA 5, 23, 24, 39, 71, 185, 194, 256
Dextromethorphan 206
DHEA 179, 191, 299
Diabetes 2, 3, 5, 6, 7, 16, 22, 23, 25, 40, 43, 46, 52, 53, 54, 58, 59, 60, 66, 69, 73, 75, 76, 91, 93, 97, 100, 109, 110, 152, 188, 189, 190, 194, 202, 203, 207, 215, 221, 230, 237, 247, 276, 278, 284
  Insulin-resistant 3, 22, 40, 43, 53, 54, 152
  Type 2 2, 5, 16, 97, 100, 109, 110, 188, 203, 215, 221, 237, 247, 278
Diagnostic and Statistical Manual of Mental Disorders 117
Diaphragmatic breaths 13
Diarrhea 40, 190, 207
Diet
  Place to start 165
DIET ALONE ALWAYS FAILS 33
Dietary fat 64, 88, 278
Dietary Fiber Causes Weight Loss 106
Dietary supplements 173, 174, 184, 300
Diethylpropion 204, 205, 306
Difficulty falling asleep 8
DNA 67, 74, 174, 222, 225, 228, 239, 240, 241, 243, 246, 305, 313, 315
Docosahexaenoic acid (DHA) 177
Dopamine antagonists 206
Dual-energy X-ray absorptiometry 23
DuBois, Eugene F. 76
Duodenum 19
Dynamic Posture Assessment 163
Dynamic stretching 121, 122, 123, 127, 128, 129, 130
  Repetitive Joint Movement 127

E

Endurance athletes 154, 178, 245

G

Gait pattern 22
GALT 221
Gastroenteritis 190
Gastrointestinal tract 94, 106, 190, 209, 219, 221
Ghrelin 16, 19, 95, 106, 166, 209, 210, 212, 253, 254, 289, 296
GI motility 19
Giuliani, Rudy 87
GLP-1 19, 92, 93, 106, 212, 289, 309
Glutamine 221, 223
Gluten 93, 94, 102
Glycemic index 62, 89
Glycogen 45, 51, 58, 61, 90, 109, 120, 166, 169
Green Tea Extract 192
Growth hormone (GH) 251, 252, 253, 254

H

Harrelson, Woody 235
Harvard Health 223
Harvard School of Public Health 85
hCG 183
HDL 55, 56, 60, 66, 88, 91, 100, 109, 170, 236
Heart attack 6, 7, 25, 86, 91, 197, 235
Heart Healthy 233
Heinon, Marina 173, 296
Hepatic portal vein 44
High blood pressure 3, 6, 25, 75, 86, 189, 226
High-carbohydrate diets 90, 98
High-fructose corn syrup 232
High glycemic foods 15, 89, 102
High-Intensity Interval Training 119
High-protein diets 166
High sugar foods 15
Hippocampal (brain) atrophy 91
Hippocampus 22, 273
HMB 167, 184
Homeostasis 48, 95, 169
Homocysteine 5, 256
Hormone replacement (HRT) 2, 8, 23, 24, 25, 27, 29, 172, 193, 199, 200, 201, 211, 212, 244, 248, 256, 303
Hyperlipidemia 22, 59, 203, 237
Hypertension 2, 3, 16, 22, 54, 58, 59, 60, 73, 91, 97, 171, 189, 201, 202, 203, 221, 230, 231, 237, 298, 301
Hypothalamus 19, 204, 207, 209, 210, 248

I

J

K

L

Metabolic syndrome 22, 55, 60, 69, 93, 94, 109, 110, 114, 290
Metformin 247, 315
Microbiome 92, 221
Minnesota starvation study 210
Minnesota Starvation Study 33
Mitochondria 50, 68, 69, 74, 110, 114, 116, 178, 189, 214, 215, 228, 246, 248, 290
Mitochondrial ATP 76
Mitochondrial density 119
Mitochondrial DNA 225
Mitochondrial theory of aging 214
Monoamine oxidase inhibitors 206
Monounsaturated fat 64, 88, 101
Monthly waist-size measurement 39
Moore, Demi 235
Morbid obesity 22
mTOR 76, 153, 213, 214, 215, 216, 247, 282, 309
mTORC1 214
mTORC2 214
mTOR kinases 213, 214
Murthy, Vivek 87
Muscle strengthening exercises 134
Mutant mitochondrial and free radical theories of aging 246
MyFitnessPal app 82
Myocardial infarction 6, 7, 86, 197, 231, 270, 299
Myofascial Release 121, 123
Myoglobin 154, 155

N

Naltrexone 207
National Academy of Sports Medicine 118, 159
National Center for Health Statistics 6, 305
National Institute of Health 21, 54, 184
National Institute of Mental Health 116
National Institute on Aging 226
National Public Radio 87
National Strength and Conditioning Association (NSCA) 159
Neurodegenerative diseases 198
Neurotransmitter GABA 200
New York Times 87, 297
Norepinephrine 51, 204, 207
NOVA 95
NPY 19
Nurses' Health Study 56, 88, 284

O

W

Y

Z

www.ingramcontent.com/pod-product-compliance
Lightning Source LLC
Chambersburg PA
CBHW050803270326
41926CB00025B/4517